Imaging in Alzheimer's Disease and Other Dementias

Guest Editor

ALISON D. MURRAY, MBChB (Hons), FRCP, FRCR

NEUROIMAGING CLINICS OF NORTH AMERICA

www.neuroimaging.theclinics.com

Consulting Editor
SURESH K. MUKHERJI, MD

February 2012 • Volume 22 • Number 1

SAUNDERS an imprint of ELSEVIER, Inc.

W.B. SAUNDERS COMPANY
A Division of Elsevier Inc.

1600 John F. Kennedy Boulevard ● Suite 1800 ● Philadelphia, Pennsylvania 19103-2899

http://www.theclinics.com

NEUROIMAGING CLINICS OF NORTH AMERICA Volume 22, Number 1
February 2012 ISSN 1052-5149, ISBN 13: 978-1-4557-4207-3

Editor: Sarah E. Barth
Developmental Editor: Donald Mumford

Neuroimaging Clinics of North America (ISSN 1052-5149) is published quarterly by Elsevier Inc., 360 Park Avenue South, New York, NY 10010-1710. Months of issue are February, May, August, and November. Business and editorial offices: 1600 John F. Kennedy Blvd., Suite 1800, Philadelphia, PA 19103-2899. Business and editorial offices: 6277 Sea Harbor Drive, Orlando, FL 32887-4800. Periodicals postage paid at New York, NY, and additional mailing offices. Subscription prices are USD 342 per year for US individuals, USD 471 per year for US institutions, USD 172 per year for US students and residents, USD 396 per year for Canadian individuals, USD 590 per year for Canadian institutions, USD 502 per year for international individuals, USD 590 per year for international institutions and USD 246 per year for Canadian and foreign students and residents. To receive student/resident rate, orders must be accompanied by name of affiliated institution, date of term, and the *signature* of program/residency coordinator on institution letterhead. Orders will be billed at individual rate until proof of status is received. Foreign air speed delivery is included in all *Clinics* subscription prices. All prices are subject to change without notice. POSTMASTER: Send address changes to *Neuroimaging Clinics of North America*, Elsevier Health Sciences Division, Subscription Customer Service, 3251 Riverport Lane, Maryland Heights, MO 63043. Telephone: 1-800-654-2452 (U.S. and Canada); 314-447-8871 (outside U.S. and Canada). Fax: 314-447-8029. E-mail: journalscustomerservice-usa@elsevier.com (for print support); journalsonlinesupport-usa@elsevier.com (for online support).

Reprints. For copies of 100 or more of articles in this publication, please contact the Commercial Reprints Department, Elsevier Inc., 360 Park Avenue South, New York, NY 10010-1710. Tel.: 212-633-3812; Fax: 212-462-1935; E-mail: reprints@elsevier.com.

Neuroimaging Clinics of North America is covered by *Excerpta Medical/EMBASE,* the RSNA Index of Imaging Literature, *MEDLINE/PubMed (Index Medicus),* MEDLINE/MEDLARS, SciSearch, Research Alert, and Neuroscience Citation Index.

Printed and bound by CPI Group (UK) Ltd, Croydon, CR0 4YY

Transferred to Digital Print 2012

GOAL STATEMENT

The goal of *Neuroimaging Clinics of North America* is to keep practicing radiologists and radiology residents up to date with current clinical practice in radiology by providing timely articles reviewing the state of the art in patient care.

ACCREDITATION

The *Neuroimaging Clinics of North America* is planned and implemented in accordance with the Essential Areas and Policies of the Accreditation Council for Continuing Medical Education (ACCME) through the joint sponsorship of the University of Virginia School of Medicine and Elsevier. The University of Virginia School of Medicine is accredited by the ACCME to provide continuing medical education for physicians.

The University of Virginia School of Medicine designates this enduring material activity for a maximum of 15 *AMA PRA Category 1 Credit*(s)™ for each issue, 60 credits per year. Physicians should claim only the credit commensurate with the extent of their participation in the activity.

The American Medical Association has determined that physicians not licensed in the US who participate in this CME enduring material activity are eligible for a maximum of 15 *AMA PRA Category 1 Credit*(s)™ for each issue, 60 credits per year.

Credit can be earned by reading the text material, taking the CME examination online at http://www.theclinics.com/home/cme, and completing the evaluation. After taking the test, you will be required to review any and all incorrect answers. Following completion of the test and evaluation, your credit will be awarded and you may print your certificate.

FACULTY DISCLOSURE/CONFLICT OF INTEREST

The University of Virginia School of Medicine, as an ACCME accredited provider, endorses and strives to comply with the Accreditation Council for Continuing Medical Education (ACCME) Standards of Commercial Support, Commonwealth of Virginia statutes, University of Virginia policies and procedures, and associated federal and private regulations and guidelines on the need for disclosure and monitoring of proprietary and financial interests that may affect the scientific integrity and balance of content delivered in continuing medical education activities under our auspices.

The University of Virginia School of Medicine requires that all CME activities accredited through this institution be developed independently and be scientifically rigorous, balanced and objective in the presentation/discussion of its content, theories and practices.

All authors/editors participating in an accredited CME activity are expected to disclose to the readers relevant financial relationships with commercial entities occurring within the past 12 months (such as grants or research support, employee, consultant, stock holder, member of speakers bureau, etc.). The University of Virginia School of Medicine will employ appropriate mechanisms to resolve potential conflicts of interest to maintain the standards of fair and balanced education to the reader. Questions about specific strategies can be directed to the Office of Continuing Medical Education, University of Virginia School of Medicine, Charlottesville, Virginia.

The faculty and staff of the University of Virginia Office of Continuing Medical Education have no financial affiliations to disclose.

The authors/editors listed below have identified no professional/financial affiliations for themselves or their spouse/ partner:
Sarah Barth, (Acquisitions Editor); Etsuko Imabayashi, MD, PhD; Stéphane Lehéricy, MD, PhD; Hiroshi Matsuda, MD, PhD; Lubdha M. Shah, MD (Test Author); Marion Smits, MD, PhD; Roger T. Staff, PhD; Maria Carmela Tartaglia, MD; John-Paul Taylor, MBBS(Hons), PhD, MRCPsych; Arthur W. Toga, PhD; Meike W. Vernooij, MD, PhD; and Lawrence J. Whalley, MD.

The authors listed below have identified the following professional/financial affiliations for themselves or their spouse/ partner:
Leonardo Cruz de Souza, MD, PhD receives speaker honraria from Lundbeck, and is an industry funded research/investigator for Roche.
Bruno Dubois, MD is on the Advisory Board for BMS, Roche, and Affiris, and is on the Speakers' Bureau for Novartis.
Charles R. Harrington, PhD owns stock in TauRx Therapeutics Ltd.
Suresh K. Mukherji, MD (Consulting Editor) is a consultant for Philips.
Alison D. Murray, MBChB (Hons), FRCP, FRCR (Guest Editor) is a patent holder with Tau Therapeutics.
John O'Brien, MA, DM, FRCPsych is a consultant for Bayer Healthcare, is on the Advisory Board for GE Healthcare and Lilly, and is on the Speakers' Board for GE Healthcare.
Marie Sarazin, MD, PhD is a consultant and is on the Advisory Board for Eisai, teaching courses for Novartis, Lundbeck, and Janssen, and is an industry funded research/investigator for Roche.

Disclosure of Discussion of Non-FDA Approved Uses for Pharmaceutical Products and/or Medical Devices
The University of Virginia School of Medicine, as an ACCME provider, requires that all faculty presenters identify and disclose any off-label uses for pharmaceutical and medical device products. The University of Virginia School of Medicine recommends that each physician fully review all the available data on new products or procedures prior to clinical use.

TO ENROLL

To enroll in the Neuroimaging Clinics of North America Continuing Medical Education program, call customer service at 1-800-654-2452 or sign up online at http://www.theclinics.com/home/cme. The CME program is available to subscribers for an additional annual fee of USD 196.

Neuroimaging Clinics of North America

THE CLINICS ARE NOW AVAILABLE ONLINE!

Access your subscription at:
www.theclinics.com

Contributors

CONSULTING EDITOR

SURESH K. MUKHERJI, MD, FACR
Professor and Chief of Neuroradiology,
and Head and Neck Radiology; Professor
of Radiology, Otolaryngology Head and Neck
Surgery, Radiation Oncology, Periodontics
and Oral Medicine, University of Michigan
Health System, Ann Arbor, Michigan

GUEST EDITOR

**ALISON D. MURRAY, MBChB (Hons),
FRCP, FRCR**
Clinical Senior Lecturer in Neuroradiology,
Aberdeen Biomedical Imaging Centre,
University of Aberdeen, Aberdeen, Scotland,
United Kingdom

AUTHORS

LEONARDO CRUZ DE SOUZA, MD, PhD
Université Pierre et Marie Curie Paris 6, Centre
de Recherche de l'Institut du Cerveau et de la
Moelle Epinière, UMR-S975; Inserm, U975;
CNRS, UMR 7225; Institut du Cerveau et de la
Moelle Epinière, ICM; Alzheimer Institute,
Research and Resource Memory Centre,
Centre de Référence des Démences Rares,
Centre de Référence maladie d'Alzheimer
jeune, AP-HP, Pitié-Salpêtrière Hospital,
Paris, France

BRUNO DUBOIS, MD
Université Pierre et Marie Curie Paris 6, Centre
de Recherche de l'Institut du Cerveau et de la
Moelle Epinière, UMR-S975; Inserm, U975;
CNRS, UMR 7225; Institut du Cerveau et de la
Moelle Epinière, ICM; Alzheimer Institute,
Research and Resource Memory Centre,
Centre de Référence des Démences Rares,
Centre de Référence maladie d'Alzheimer
jeune, AP-HP, Pitié-Salpêtrière Hospital,
Paris, France

CHARLES R. HARRINGTON, PhD
Senior Research Fellow, Division of Applied
Health Sciences, School of Medicine and
Dentistry, Institute of Medical Sciences,
University of Aberdeen, Aberdeen, Scotland,
United Kingdom

ETSUKO IMABAYASHI, MD, PhD
Assistant Professor, Department of Nuclear
Medicine, Saitama Medical University
International Medical Center, Hidaka,
Saitama, Japan

STÉPHANE LEHÉRICY, MD, PhD
Université Pierre et Marie Curie Paris 6, Centre
de Recherche de l'Institut du Cerveau et de la
Moelle Epinière, UMR-S975; Inserm, U975;
CNRS, UMR 7225; Institut du Cerveau et de la
Moelle Epinière, ICM; Centre de Neuroimagerie
de Recherche – CENIR and Department of
Neuroradiology, Pitié-Salpêtrière Hospital,
Paris, France

HIROSHI MATSUDA, MD, PhD
Professor, Department of Nuclear Medicine, Saitama Medical University International Medical Center, Hidaka, Saitama, Japan

JOHN O'BRIEN, MA, DM, FRCPsych
Professor of Old Age Psychiatry, Institute for Ageing and Health, Wolfson Research Centre, Campus for Ageing and Vitality, Newcastle University, Newcastle Upon Tyne, United Kingdom

MARIE SARAZIN, MD, PhD
Université Pierre et Marie Curie Paris 6, Centre de Recherche de l'Institut du Cerveau et de la Moelle Epinière, UMR-S975; Inserm, U975; CNRS, UMR 7225; Institut du Cerveau et de la Moelle Epinière, ICM; Alzheimer Institute, Research and Resource Memory Centre, Centre de Référence des Démences Rares, Centre de Référence maladie d'Alzheimer jeune, AP-HP, Pitié-Salpêtrière Hospital, Paris, France

MARION SMITS, MD, PhD
Neuroradiologist and Assistant Professor in Radiology, Department of Radiology, Erasmus MC University Medical Center, Rotterdam, The Netherlands

ROGER T. STAFF, PhD
Aberdeen Royal Infirmary, Department of Bio-Medical Physics, NHS-Grampian and the University of Aberdeen, Foresterhill, Aberdeen, Scotland, United Kingdom

MARIA CARMELA TARTAGLIA, MD
Assistant Professor, Tanz Centre for Research in Neurodegenerative Diseases, University of Toronto, Toronto, Ontario, Canada

JOHN-PAUL TAYLOR, MBBS(Hons), PhD, MRCPsych
Wellcome Intermediate Clinical Fellow and Honorary Consultant in Old Age Psychiatry, Institute for Ageing and Health, Wolfson Research Centre, Campus for Ageing and Vitality, Newcastle University, Newcastle Upon Tyne, United Kingdom

ARTHUR W. TOGA, PhD
Laboratory of Neuro Imaging, Department of Neurology, David Geffen School of Medicine at UCLA, Los Angeles, California

MEIKE W. VERNOOIJ, MD, PhD
Neuroradiologist and Assistant Professor in Radiology, Department of Radiology; Assistant Professor in Epidemiology, Department of Epidemiology, Erasmus MC University Medical Center, Rotterdam, The Netherlands

LAWRENCE J. WHALLEY, MD
Crombie Ross Professor of Mental Health, Institute of Applied Health Sciences, School of Medicine and Dentistry, University of Aberdeen, Aberdeen, Scotland, United Kingdom

Contents

> There are well-established differences in dementia incidence between communities and within communities over time. In part, these differences may be attributable to local improvements in dementia diagnosis and classification. Nevertheless, there are grounds for cautious optimism that there have been slight, but significant, recent reductions in dementia incidence. Possible causes include public health measures to reduce mortality attributable to stroke and heart disease, improved nutrition, and greater personal wealth. A life-course approach to dementia pathophysiology may help to elucidate the nature and timing of interventions that might delay dementia onset.

> Neurofibrillary pathology in Alzheimer's disease consists of paired helical filaments comprising tau protein. This pathology is correlated with dementia, but can appear in the first two decades of life. Extracellular amyloid β-protein arises through proteolytic processing of a transmembrane precursor, which involves the action of several enzymes. Mutations in the genes for the precursor and presenilin proteins accelerate the deposition of Aβ. Tau mutations cause other tauopathies in the absence of amyloid deposition, indicating that amyloid deposition is not a prerequisite for dementia. An improved understanding of Alzheimer's disease awaits to be obtained by molecular imaging of these pathologies.

> In contrast with the previous criteria published in 1984 by the National Institute of Neurological and Communicative Disorders and Stroke and the Alzheimer's Disease and Related Disorders Association, the new criteria proposed in 2007 incorporated in the diagnostic framework the use of biomarkers that are able to assess the underlying pathophysiologic mechanism. The combination of clinical and biologic approaches makes a diagnosis of Alzheimer's disease possible before the dementia stage. The core clinical criteria continue to be the cornerstone of the diagnosis in clinical practice, but biomarker evidence is expected to enhance the specificity for the diagnosis of Alzheimer's disease.

> The role of structural neuroimaging in the diagnosis of Alzheimer's disease (AD) is becoming increasingly important. As a consequence, a basic understanding of

what are normal brain changes in aging is key to be able to recognize what is abnormal. The first part of this article discusses normal versus pathologic brain aging, focusing on qualitative and quantitative magnetic resonance (MR) imaging markers. In the second part, the role of MR imaging in the (differential) diagnosis of AD is reviewed.

This article reviews current amyloid positron emission tomography (PET) imaging with particular attention to Pittsburgh compound-B (PiB), the most extensively investigated and validated tracer. PiB specifically binds to fibrillar β-amyloid deposits such as those found in the cerebral cortex and striatum. PiB-PET imaging is a sensitive and specific biologic marker for underlying amyloid deposition, which is an early event on the path to dementia. Amyloid imaging in healthy controls and patients with mild cognitive impairment may detect those at high risk of future Alzheimer's disease, identifying them as candidates for early preventive measures if and when they become available.

Dementia with Lewy bodies (DLB) is a relative newcomer to the field of late-life dementia. Although a diversity of imaging methodologies is now available for the study of dementia, these have been applied most often to Alzheimer's disease (AD). Studies on DLB, although fewer, have yielded fascinating and important insights into the underlying pathophysiology of this condition and allowed clinical differentiation of DLB from other dementias. Imaging research on DLB has had significant ramifications in terms of raising the profile of DLB and helping define it as a distinctive and separate disease entity from AD.

Frontotemporal dementia (FTD) describes a group of clinical syndromes united by underlying frontotemporal lobar degeneration (FTLD) pathology. The clinical syndromes associated with FTLD are heterogeneous and are based on whether the patients present with behavioral, language, or motor impairments. FTLD is at the center of a paradigm shift in neurodegenerative diseases, with thought being given at diagnosis of underlying disease. There is pathologic heterogeneity of certain clinical syndromes such as behavioral variant FTD. Differentiation between the proteinopathies will become imperative as protein-specific treatments become available. This review provides an overview of FTLD, with an update of recent discoveries.

Reserve refers to the brain's ability to cope with increasing damage. There is no direct measure of reserve, but it is commonly reflected in the literature by proxies such as brain volume, head size, education, occupation, socioeconomic status, and mental and physical engagement. This article provides an overview of the concepts and applications being used to explore reserve, and discusses how these empiric proxies of reserve, their hypothesized biological mechanisms, and the apparent protection from age-related disease are connected.

Rapid advances in neuroimaging and cyberinfrastructure technologies have brought explosive growth in the Web-based warehousing, availability, and accessibility of imaging data on a variety of neurodegenerative and neuropsychiatric disorders and conditions. There has been a prolific development and emergence of complex computational infrastructures that serve as repositories of databases and provide critical functionalities such as sophisticated image analysis algorithm pipelines and powerful three-dimensional visualization and statistical tools. The statistical and operational advantages of collaborative, distributed team science in the form of multisite consortia push this approach in a diverse range of population-based investigations.

Foreword

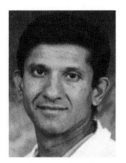

Suresh K. Mukherji, MD
Consulting Editor

The one thing none of us can escape is "Father Time"! As a result, the fastest growing segment of neuroimaging is dementia. The current prevalence of dementia is anticipated to double every 20 years as people live longer. All radiologists will be aware of a steady rise in the number of requests for brain imaging in the elderly (which is defined as 10 years older than me!). Neuroimaging in dementia is recommended by most clinical guidelines and its role has traditionally been to exclude a mass lesion, rather than to support a specific diagnosis.

Dr Allison Murray has done a wonderful job in creating a very special edition on dementia imaging. In this edition, she has brought together a very experienced group of authors to cover a broad range of topics in dementia imaging that include Alzheimer's disease (AD), frontotemporal dementia, and Lewy body dementia. She also includes specific articles on AD that include epidemiology, molecular basis, diagnostic criteria, and molecular imaging in AD. This issue is truly a state-of-the-art contribution that will help us in our clinical practice and advance the field of dementia imaging. I am very grateful to Dr Murray and all of her contributors for the tremendous efforts they have invested in creating such an outstanding edition.

Suresh K. Mukherji, MD
Department of Radiology
University of Michigan Health System
1500 East Medical Center
Ann Arbor, MI 48109-0030, USA

E-mail address:
mukherji@med.umich.edu

doi:10.1016/j.nic.2011.12.002

neuroimaging.theclinics.com

Preface

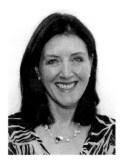

Alison D. Murray, MBChB (Hons), FRCP, FRCR
Guest Editor

Dementia is a massive and increasing global problem, with the current prevalence anticipated to double every 20 years as people live longer. Neuroimaging in dementia is recommended by most clinical guidelines and its role has traditionally been to exclude a mass lesion, rather than to support a specific diagnosis. All radiologists will be aware of a steady rise in the number of requests for brain imaging in elderly people, but what can imaging reliably tell us and what kind of imaging should we use? In affluent societies we now have a range of structural and molecular brain imaging techniques at our disposal, with specific ligands and sophisticated image analysis techniques now available for clinical use. However, we have difficulty justifying which patients to scan, which modality to use, and when imaging patients with dementia is most useful. We know that Alzheimer's disease is the most common neuropathology contributing to a diagnosis of dementia but we also know from large post-mortem studies that most brain pathology in those who have died with a diagnosis of dementia is mixed. Thus understanding different diseases that can cause dementia, how these co-exist or interact, and appreciating that not all dementia is Alzheimer's disease is important. Equally important is the awareness of individual differences in response to a neuropathological burden and what factors provide "cognitive reserve" or resilience against dementia that might be maximized to reduce or postpone its impact.

This edition draws together contributions from experts in their fields in nine articles. First, Lawrence Whalley sets the scene with a review of current knowledge on the epidemiology of dementia and describes factors that increase and decrease risk. The molecular pathology of Alzheimer's disease is described in detail in the second article by Charlie Harrington. In the third article, Marie Sarazin and colleagues provide a comprehensive description of the research criteria for a diagnosis of Alzheimer's disease and illustrate the important role imaging now has in detecting the disease before the patient has become demented. In the fourth article, Meike Vernooij and Marion Smits detail the structural neuroimaging correlates of normal aging and of Alzheimer's disease, indicating the variety of MRI findings in the aging brain that are associated with cognitive decline. Hiroshi Matsuda and Etsuko Imabayashi discuss molecular imaging in Alzheimer's disease, concentrating on evidence for the current role of Pittsburgh Compound B in article 5. In the sixth article, Jean-Paul Taylor and John O'Brien cover the clinical and neuroimaging features of dementia with Lewy bodies, an increasingly recognized and important cause of dementia, and illustrate that it may be just as relevant to image the heart, rather than the head. Carmella Tartaglia describes the neuropathology and imaging features of different diseases that cause frontotemporal dementia in the seventh article and illustrates how advances in understanding of the molecular pathology of these diseases are changing our understanding of neurodegenerative disease in general. Cerebral reserve is reviewed in article 8 by Roger Staff, who illustrates the importance of understanding and quantifying reserve in cognitive aging research and how, because of reserve, imaging can provide a more accurate measure of the neuropathological burden than clinical assessment. Finally, in the last article, Arthur Toga describes how large databases, such as the Alzheimer's Disease Neuroimaging Initiative, have brought about a new era of collaborative, interdisciplinary research that promises neuroimaging as a valid outcome measure in clinical trials of future treatments.

This is a fast moving and exciting time for neuroimaging in dementia research and clinical practice.

Alison D. Murray, MBChB (Hons), FRCP, FRCR
Aberdeen Biomedical Imaging Centre
University of Aberdeen
Aberdeen AB25 2ZD, UK

E-mail address:
a.d.murray@abdn.ac.uk

Spatial Distribution and Secular Trends in the Epidemiology of Alzheimer's Disease

Lawrence J. Whalley, MD

KEYWORDS

- Geography • Secular trends • Diagnosis • Nutrition
- Vascular risk • Stroke • Fetal origins of adult disease
- Life-course methods

Key Points: ALZHEIMER'S DISEASE EPIDEMIOLOGY

1. There is nonrandom distribution of dementia incidence in space and time.

2. International comparisons are needed to estimate the current and future dementia burden in developed and developing countries.

3. In developed countries, there is some evidence that dementia incidence is decreasing, and this may be attributable to public health measures to reduce vascular disease and/or greater personal resources to buffer the effects of dementia.

4. Nutritional epidemiology is relevant to understanding how and why dementia incidence might vary in space and time. This is true of folate/vitamin B_{12} metabolism and, possibly, dietary fish oil.

5. A life-course approach to understanding how and when risk factors increase susceptibility to vascular disease is relevant to late-life dementia. This approach may identify epigenetic pathways that involve both environmental and molecular genetic factors.

There are many excellent recent reviews on the epidemiology of Alzheimer's disease (AD). Almost all evaluate evidence for the role of specific factors that increase the risk of AD[1] or, less often, discuss the effects of risk factors that might offer some protection against AD.[2] This article does not examine these issues but focuses on trends in the spatial and secular incidence of AD that have remained neglected by reviewers. Related questions arising from the genetic epidemiology of AD, although relevant when international comparisons are considered, are in their infancy and are outside the scope of this review. However, 2 points are relevant and are listed here for completeness.

First, at one time it seemed that epidemiologic studies in dementia would be superseded by advances in laboratory molecular genetics. Supported by identification of genetic mutations in early onset AD (EOAD), claims were made that the causes of AD, irrespective of age at onset, were genetic and that these would soon be remediable. So far, among many putative associations only *APOEε4* has remained a well-established genetic susceptibility factor for late-onset AD (LOAD).[3] Molecular genetic research programs can deploy large-scale detection techniques using genome-wide association study methods. These powerful methods detect many genes each of small effect and results so far are

Funding support: Supported in part by Alzheimer Research UK.

Institute of Applied Health Sciences, School of Medicine and Dentistry, University of Aberdeen, Polwarth Building, Aberdeen AB25 2ZH, UK

E-mail address: l.j.whalley@abdn.ac.uk

Neuroimag Clin N Am 22 (2012) 1–10

doi:10.1016/j.nic.2011.11.002

promising. However, convincing replication of findings in LOAD remains elusive and, at least for some time, a considered combination of molecular genetic and epidemiologic methods will continue to be used to unravel the complex multifactorial causes of AD.[4] To date, no evidence relevant to understanding genetic sources of differences between geographic areas has been presented.

Second, epidemiologic data cannot be assumed to be transferable across cultures or to be stable within 1 culture over time. However, what seems like a major potential source of error can become a strength and it is here that spatial epidemiology is most helpful. Apparent inconsistencies in cross-cultural epidemiologic observational data provide clues to the complex multifactorial nature of the dementias. When well-defined populations differ significantly from others in patterns of AD incidence, their genetic structures and environmental exposures become topics of intense scrutiny. The best-known example is found among the Chamarro people of the Pacific Island of Guam who suffer from a complex syndrome with features of Parkinson disease, AD, and motor neuron disease (the Parkinson-dementia complex of Guam) but for whom there is no clear-cut evidence for either a genetic or environmental cause.[5]

DEMENTIA DIAGNOSIS AND CLASSIFICATION

Secular trends and spatial distributions of AD are relevant to understanding how multiple causal factors might influence life-course pathways toward AD.[6] To become a case of dementia, an individual must cross thresholds of loss of cognitive performance and activities of daily living, and should show worsening progression from a premorbid (ie, original) level of mental performance. These thresholds are open to individual variation. People of higher socioeconomic status who have strong family support and who can retain sufficient mental flexibility to compensate for early deficits attributable to the presence of brain pathology present to health services later in the course of their dementia.[7] At presentation, these individuals often show a greater degree of brain pathology than those who do not have similar support or advantageous socioeconomic circumstances.[8] Therefore, it follows that, when there are improvements in the material well-being of a society, when measures are in place to enhance family and community support, the apparent incidence of dementia might decline. Accurate dementia case ascertainment should continue to rely on prospective longitudinal studies with access to a wide range of data sources relevant to both hospital-treated cases and those who remain in the community and do not enter the hospital system.

These considerations weaken the preconception that a simple mechanistic model of dementia onset, with gold standard criteria for case recognition, suffices for all individuals with dementia. In turn, acceptance of sources of individual variation indicates that, in some instances, certain putative risk factors for dementia identified in observational studies might not be determinants of dementia but consequences of case-finding methodology. A good example of the steps needed to identify and allow for these effects was provided by a ground-breaking cross-cultural study.[9–11]

During the second half of the last century, consistent measures of the incidence and prevalence of late-onset dementias were gradually established. Using harmonized diagnostic criteria and acceptable survey methods, findings from pioneering European studies in Scandinavia, the United Kingdom, Italy, and Holland[12–15] were used to inform public policy and social and biomedical research. Within the broad grouping of the late-onset dementias, and encouraged by progress in neurochemical studies, governments and the pharmaceutical industry began to focus on AD almost to the exclusion of other forms of dementia. The public and press became aware of AD as a major cause of disability and premature death that was seriously underreported and had remained a neglected research topic. Opinion leaders emphasized that the burgeoning epidemic of AD would become the single greatest threat to the maintenance of health care and living standards of old people, with great potential to jeopardize the capacity of developed countries to maintain satisfactory standards of health care and social support for all sections of society.[16] Urgent concern about the implications of a silent dementia epidemic is, with hindsight, now recognized as the first tangible benefit of more than 25 years of intense epidemiologic research in dementia.

Although broadly similar estimates of the incidence and prevalence of AD are now widely accepted, there are some caveats. The first is that research methods have differed between localities and over time. Specifically, European investigators pioneered diagnostic procedures based on standardized psychiatric interviews and were greatly influenced by the success of the UK-US diagnostic project for which an interview-based method[17] (The Present State Examination [PSE]) amenable to the application of computerized diagnostic algorithms was developed. The PSE was founded on precise definitions of psychopathology that would discriminate most efficiently between functional psychoses, specifically schizophrenia, and the affective psychoses. Systematic questions posed by trained interviewers (who did not need to be clinicians) contained elements of each definition to determine the presence of a symptom or sign of disorder, its severity, and its duration. The PSE did not deal adequately with the dementias and Copeland and colleagues[18] addressed this deficiency by applying the PSE format to dementia diagnosis, leading to the development of the Geriatric Mental State (GMS) Examination. As with the PSE, computer-based algorithms provided classifications of the mental disorders of late life, each of which could be validated against clinical examinations that included data from a clinical history, from informants, and, where indicated, from a limited neurologic examination.

These semistructured interviews represented a major improvement on previous attempts at case finding in epidemiologic studies of dementia. Although most often used in a single interview, the interviews could be used in 2 or more phases in longitudinal studies of dementia incidence. During this early phase of development of diagnostic criteria for AD for use in epidemiologic studies, great care was taken to distinguish between dementias of presumed vascular origin and dementia without evidence of cerebrovascular disease. A simple checklist[19] had been devised from criteria listed in standard textbooks and provided a total score to represent the presence of cortical infarcts. In large part, this approach was based on the idea that detection of large cortical infarcts supported a diagnosis of multi-infarct dementia and allowed for minor cerebrovascular involvement with some AD features but, if there was no evidence of cerebrovascular disease, then an AD diagnosis was likely. The diagnosis of AD was, therefore, made largely by exclusion of other causes of dementia, principally vascular dementias.

In the United States, dementia researchers developed a second approach that is now popular in European studies, probably because it makes better use of the wide range of possible data sources relevant to a dementia diagnosis. The US approach accepted that, in the absence of valid and reliable diagnostic biomarkers to detect the presence of dementia or any of its subtypes, and faced by variations between clinicians in the detection and recording of diagnostic features, a consensus group drawn from relevant disciplines (eg, psychiatry, neurology, clinical psychology, neuroimaging, neuropathology) could achieve agreement on diagnostic classification in the absence of gold standard biomarkers.[20] This approach allowed for variation in mental state over time and the presence of vascular lesions, and provided a counterbalance to the tendency for the application of diagnostic procedures to become idiosyncratic when reliance was placed solely on a single individual repeatedly applying the same criteria to datasets of uneven quality. The US approach was particularly notable for its clear recommendations that certain cognitive deficits were more often found in early AD (eg, dyspraxia) than in other dementias. Advantages of the prevailing US approach included the opportunity to examine relationships between acute cerebrovascular events as triggers for the gradual onset of dementia of the Alzheimer type,[21] whereas, at that time, the European approach would most likely have categorized any subsequent dementia as cerebrovascular in origin. The consensus approach also identified opportunities to improve dementia diagnoses using biomarkers.[22]

The US consensual diagnostic approach seems also to deal appropriately with the contribution of individual differences in the capacity to cope with or adjust for the presence of dementia pathology. This last is not a trivial point: the capacity of an individual to cope with a dementia disorder may depend on personal attributes loosely labeled resilience, but more precisely may be understood as aspects of intelligence, a socially engaged lifestyle, and a preference for mentally effortful recreational pursuits. The idea that an individual possesses a quantifiable cognitive reserve[23] to mitigate the effects of neuropathology (arising from dementia or brain damage incurred through stroke or trauma) is widely discussed and is supported by the repeated observation that there is not a direct relationship between the degree of brain pathology and the severity of clinical features of dementia. From an epidemiologic perspective, the positive contributions of cognitive reserve that could buffer the effects of AD neuropathology suggest a basic distinction between those factors that increase AD risk and those that decrease it, perhaps through neuroprotective mechanisms.

THE GEOGRAPHY OF DEMENTIA

Shared environmental exposures and nongenetic transmission of disease are closely related to detection of spatial proximity. Observational studies of this type often assume that risk of disease is greater if people at increased risk are closely related in space and time. The basic approach in spatial epidemiology is to examine maps of disease distributions and/or secular trends in the incidence of a disease. Beyond this basic idea lies a major problem of testing a statistical hypothesis. The typical aim is to identify clusters of disease, but these aims rarely extend to explicit causal inferences being drawn with confidence from the data. However, in terms of public understanding of disease risk, maps provide an accessible method of presenting otherwise difficult-to-understand scientific evidence in support of a particular estimation of disease risk.

The prevailing research strategy in the epidemiology of LOAD is to study multiple risk factors in samples at risk of LOAD on grounds of age and the presence or absence of specific risk factors (eg, family history of dementia). Population samples are usually drawn from well-defined areas with known demographics. It is especially helpful if exposures to dementia risk or neuroprotective factors have already been established in the population. A good example of this approach is provided by studies that explored the possible benefits and timing of nonsteroidal antiinflammatory agents (NSAIDs) in the prevention of AD.[24] Table 1 is adapted from population-based cross-sectional studies at 11 study sites[10] and summarizes current estimates of the prevalence of dementia adjusted for differences in the age and sex distribution of local populations. This type of study is an excellent example of the research methods required in spatial epidemiology to understand how dementia might present at different sites, how diagnostic practices might influence findings, and how levels of dementia-related disability are important. The investigators needed to devise methods to adjust for survival differences, socioeconomic factors, and variations in education and health service provision between geographic regions to obtain reliable estimates of dementia prevalence in each study locality.

International studies also support the proposal that dementia prevalence varies between geographic regions, and encourages the view that environmental exposures contribute to dementia.[25] Among these studies, comparisons between African Americans living in Indianapolis (IN) and the indigenous Yoruba living in and around Ibadan in Nigeria provide compelling evidence that these international differences between populations are not spurious and require explanation.[26,27] The Ibadan-Indianapolis studies stimulated useful discussion about the genetic structure of African American and native Nigerian populations and how intergenerational continuities of poverty and poor diet could have affected African Americans to a greater extent than native Nigerians, and stimulated a search for sources of geographic difference in dementia risk. The heuristic value of these comparisons has several possible explanations:

a. More stressful urban life of African Americans
b. Lower intensity and shorter duration of formal schooling among rural African Americans[28]
c. Exposure in urban United States to pollutant neurotoxins (eg, atmospheric lead)
d. A Western diet that is calorie rich and nutrient poor
e. An increased risk of abnormal age-related glucose metabolism and type II diabetes
f. Greater use of alcohol and tobacco among African Americans
g. Better diet of native Nigerians, with fewer calories, more fresh fruit and vegetables, little red meat, and more fish
h. Differences in intracerebral cholesterol metabolism between Nigerians and African Americans.[29]

Scottish studies on the geographic distribution of EOAD support the view that EOAD distribution is nonrandom.[30–33] Clusters of cases were found in areas of Scotland associated with coal mining at the time of birth of EOAD cases. Kinship analyses of these clusters[34,35] suggested that genetic relatedness did not explain these areas of high EOAD density.

To understand environments within which an individual develops and loses cognitive competencies, it is helpful to apply research methods that can distinguish between different components of

Table 1
Prevalence of dementia by geographic region and in comparison with prevalence estimates from a meta-analysis of European sites

Study Sites	Standardized Prevalence (%)	SMR (EURODEM)[a]
Latin America (urban)	4.6	80 (70–91)
Latin America (rural)	1.5	27 (16–41)
China (urban)	3.0	57 (36–86)
China (rural)	2.4	56 (32–91)
India (urban)	0.9	22 (7–41)
India (rural)	0.8	18 (5–34)

Abbreviations: EURODEM, European Community Concerted Action on the Epidemiology of Dementia; SMR, standardized morbidity ratio.

[a] SMR is obtained by applying estimates derived from pooled European surveys (EURODEM) to the samples recruited at each of the listed study sites. An SMR of 100 implies that the observed number of dementia cases agrees with the number expected in that sample using EURODEM estimates; an SMR less than 100 implies that the prevalence is lower than would be expected in a European sample with the same age and sex distribution.

Data from Llibre Rodriguez JJ, Ferri CP, Acosta D, et al. Prevalence of dementia in Latin America, India, and China: a population-based cross-sectional survey. Lancet 2008;372(9637):464–74.

the environment that are relevant to cognitive maturation and decline. This distinction can be achieved by arranging environmental influences in a hierarchy based on the size of their effects at different points in the life course and judgments about the relative importance of specific timing of exposures (critical periods). These methods of life-course research in aging research and in the epidemiology of diseases of late life (including the dementias) are in the first phase of construction. Life-course theory has the potential to draw together apparently diverse contributions identified in epidemiologic studies concerning the causes of late-onset dementias including AD. The application of life-course methodology to different geographic settings has the potential to show how childhood experiences can modify the risk of late-onset dementia.[6]

SECULAR TRENDS IN THE INCIDENCE OF DEMENTIA

Dementia was recognized in antiquity but was not considered a major public health problem until the latter part of the twentieth century. Until about 1975, most senile dementia was attributed to hardening of the arteries of the brain, and the diagnosis of AD was reserved for rare forms of early onset (presenile) dementia that were often familial. The discovery of neurochemical abnormalities in AD consolidated the view, put forward from about 1955, that Alzheimer neuropathology accounted for more than 50% of senile dementia. Eventually, this view prevailed over the idea that cerebrovascular disease was more important largely because, at the time, it seemed that, in a manner akin to Parkinson disease, if AD could become a neurotransmitter deficiency disorder, then it could potentially become treatable using therapies that replaced or mimicked the transmitter deficiency. This change did not obviate the inclusion of risk factors for vascular disease among studies of causes in AD and, as discussed later, the vascularization of AD has proceeded steadily for 3 decades since the discovery of the cholinergic deficit in AD.

Community-based studies have consistently shown that the neuropathologic findings among those dying with a clinical dementia syndrome were typically mixed, with features of both AD and cerebrovascular disease neuropathology.[36] Rather than claiming that clinical dementia can be confidently attributed to either AD or cerebrovascular disease, many now argue that these 2 types of pathology are frequently detectable in the aged brain and that the rate of progress to dementia is determined by factors (some genetic, some environmental) that differ between individuals, to the net effect that both types of pathology contribute additively to the dementia syndrome.

These observations are relevant to understanding secular trends in the incidence of dementia. If it were accepted that vascular risk factors are implicated among the causes of AD, then it is reasonable to hypothesize that reduction of exposure to vascular risk (eg, public health measures to limit tobacco smoking, encouragement to exercise, and to be moderate in dietary habits and alcohol intake) should lead to a reduction in AD incidence. To date, there are few reports that investigate this proposal. However, in a landmark study, Rocca and colleagues[37] describe 4 observational studies, including their own, that together approximate to a US national picture of changes in AD incidence. The studies came from Rochester, Minnesota (1975–1994)[37]; the Chicago Health and Aging Project (1997–2008)[38,39]; Indianapolis (1992 and 2001)[40]; and the National Health and Retirement Study (1993 and 2002).[41] The 4 studies present different approaches to the detection of trends in dementia incidence, each providing data relevant to identification and management of those at risk of dementia through description of factors that seemed influential in modifying that risk over time. Their aims included recognition of determinants of elements of social and health care of the elderly that would inform health planning in the twenty-first century.

Rocca and colleagues[37] commented on improvements in mortality of the national US population that could be associated confidently with interventions to control hypertension, hyperlipidemia, and abnormal glucose metabolism. These reductions in mortality caused by stroke and heart disease seemed sufficient to argue that dementia incidence should have fallen in step with these measures to improve public health. Their findings were largely negative in the Minnesota, Indiana, and Illinois studies but the National Health and Retirement Study provided grounds for cautious optimism. This large national study found (using neuropsychological measures without reliance on detection of dementia caseness) that the proportion of old people who developed cognitive impairment was significantly less in the later-born birth cohorts than in the older individuals. Such improvements over time are considered to be associated with longer duration of education and greater net worth (wealth) of the later-born old people. Rocca and colleagues[37] also noted that worsening of national health statistics linked to growing numbers of obese and poorly controlled hypertensive individuals would potentially have countered any improvements in dementia incidence and that these effects may be subject to local variations to a greater extent than in the National Health and Retirement Study.

COULD NUTRITION EXPLAIN VARIATION IN DEMENTIA INCIDENCE?

Secular trends in dementia incidence could be closely related to the nutritional origins of individual differences in rates of biological aging, how these evolved, and how changing environments could have affected aging. The basis of this inference is that, like many of the cancers and atherosclerotic disorders, AD is an age-dependent condition,[42] and it implicates biological aging as a necessary precondition of the pathogenesis of AD. Theories of biological aging could therefore be relevant to understanding the neurobiology of age-related cognitive decline and AD. This view is supported by stronger associations between cognitive decline and biological measures of aging than with chronologic age.[43] However, firm links between inception of AD and rates of biological aging have not been established. For example, there are no associations between AD and other age-dependent conditions (eg, osteoporosis, some cancers, and chronic obstructive pulmonary disease[44]).

Interest in nutritional sources of variation in dementia incidence is related to the possibility that biological aging reflects the accumulation of damage to large bioregulatory molecules that are inefficiently replaced or repaired. This type of age-related damage is attributable to oxidative stress, in which excessive free radicals of oxygen are generated and antioxidant defenses are insufficient to counter their effects.[45] Antioxidant defenses comprise 2 elements: enzymatic (eg, superoxide dismutase) or nonenzymatic circulating micronutrients (eg, vitamin C).[46] This line of reasoning has supported nutritional surveys among those at risk of dementia by reason of increasing age. So far, no convincing epidemiologic evidence has been provided to establish an important role for specific antioxidant micronutrients in the pathogenesis of AD. Issues of reverse causality are sometimes inadequately addressed so that it is not possible to distinguish the pathway from a poor diet to AD from that followed when impaired cognition in early dementia impairs the ability to obtain and prepare a nutritious diet.

However, when dietary patterns are investigated, the overall intake of a diet rich in antioxidants and fish with modest amounts of red meat and red wine (The Mediterranean Diet) seems to have advantages compared with a typical Western diet with more calories, fewer antioxidants, more saturated fats, and greater consumption of beer and spirits.[47] In conjunction with genetic variation in response to specific dietary micronutrients, these nutritional data could provide explanations for the geographic variation in dementia incidence. A major research effort is currently underway to examine the sources of variation between countries and cultures in the incidence of AD. When considered alongside migration studies of the Japanese from Japan, from Hawaii, the northwestern United States, and Brazil, or African Americans from Indianapolis, there is a strong case to pursue these lines of enquiry because they seem likely to have wider relevance.

The possible role of obesity in midlife has been explored is some surveys, and there are important statistical issues when so many risk factors for vascular disorders are highly intercorrelated in Western societies. Obesity, hypertension, abnormal glucose metabolism, and hyperlipidemia frequently coexist, sometimes in association with a sedentary lifestyle, smoking, and low socioeconomic status.[48] Nevertheless, careful analysis of these factors present in midlife has separated their diverse influences and identified an important role for obesity, in conjunction with the metabolic syndrome,[49] as independent contributors to AD risk.

The importance of diet and intake of specific micronutrients in brain development is well established. A sufficiency of calories and a mixed balanced diet ensures adequate growth and cognitive development that, in conjunction with positive parenting, optimizes child development. These same factors are also important in later life such that malnutrition is a major risk factor for increased disability and disease morbidity among old people. These ill effects also include increased risks of cognitive impairment, so nutritional assessment has become a key component of evaluation in old-age medicine and in the dementia clinic. However, the scientific basis for nutritional interventions to promote retention of cognitive function in late life, or even prevent or delay dementia onset, remains uncertain. Nevertheless, there are 2 pertinent examples from studies on the nutritional epidemiology of dementia that merit comment.

Homocysteine

A good case can be made that homocysteine (HCY) increases the risk of cognitive decline and AD. The evidence from observational studies, with 1 exception,[50] shows that increased plasma HCY concentrations are linked to increased dementia risk.[51] Intervention studies intended to lower HCY concentrations have not, so far, provided evidence that this strategy can reduce dementia risk.[52] Folate deficiency at the time of conception has been linked to hypomethylation of noncoding DNA that regulates the expression of genes critical to specific times during neurodevelopment. Plausibly, abnormal DNA methylation could modify the risk of adult disease.[52] This points to several possible pathways, all involving folate/homocysteine metabolism, that could increase dementia risk[6] and, when dietary availability of folate varies between localities or over time, might explain geographic and/or secular variation in dementia incidence.

Docosohexanoic Acid and Eicosohexanoic Acid

The dietary intake of marine oils rich in the omega 3 essential fatty acids docosohexanoic acid (DHA) and eicosopentanoic acid (EPA) are linked to improved health, with claims of specific benefits for respiratory function, cardiovascular disease,

and inflammatory disorders.[53] The benefits for central nervous system function include greater intellectual development and retention of cognitive function in late life among breast-fed infants (human breast milk is replete with DHA and EPA, whereas formula feed prepared from cows' milk is not) and in epidemiologic studies of cognitive aging and dementia. Intervention studies testing cognitive benefits of DHA and EPA supplementation have not supported these claims.[54] Nevertheless, studies that compare dementia incidence between Asian communities with high dietary fish oil intake and those with predominantly inland (pastoral) dietary habits, where oily fish is unavailable, are currently underway.

SYNTHESIS

A diet deficient in essential micronutrients (eg, specific vitamins or antioxidants) might increase AD risk and could explain why specific locations or birth epochs could be associated with increased

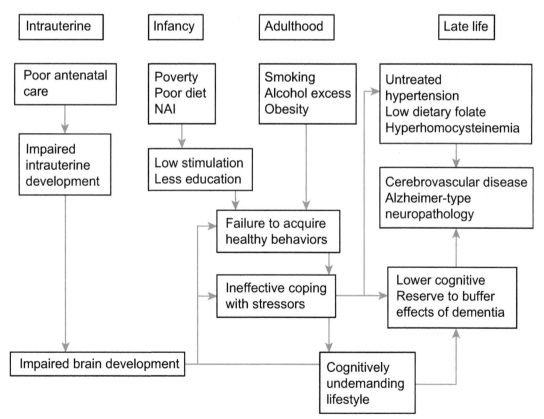

Fig. 1. A life-course approach to the epidemiology of AD showing the timing of major influences on cognitive development, the acquisition of unhealthy behaviors, and major dietary factors that increase dementia risk in late life and others that may protect against or slow the onset of dementia. NAI, non-accidental injury. (*Adapted from* Whalley LJ, Dick FD, McNeill G. A life-course approach to the aetiology of late-onset dementias. Lancet Neurol 2006;5(1):88; with permission.)

AD incidence. However, no consensus has been reached on these topics. There remains insufficient convincing data from randomized controlled trials to show that dietary supplementation is linked to better retention of cognitive abilities in late life or the prevention/delay of dementia onset.

Data on geographic distribution of dementia are strongly suggestive of risk factors common to dementia and stroke.[55] When taken together with observations of associations between vascular risk factors and both inception and survival in dementia,[56,57] the role of vascular risk factors in the pathophysiology of AD is further strengthened and becomes worthy of enquiry. The life-course approach to understanding how factors that increase susceptibility to late-life vascular disease provides a useful model, illustrated in **Fig. 1**, which represents a provisional synthesis of epidemiologic observations in dementia. It has some potential to identify time points when the risk of dementia might be lessened and draws attention to the possibility that control of vascular risk factors in midlife might reduce AD risk.

In this article, some of the main concepts and the implications of nonrandom spatial distribution and secular trends of dementia are reviewed and advanced as the basis for further discussion. The most important are (1) the strength of evidence for international differences in dementia distribution; (2) the need to investigate and monitor changes over time in dementia incidence, partly because of covariation with reductions in vascular disease but also because, as societies become more affluent, so their dementia risk might increase; (3) the need to model the pathophysiology of AD to inform how dementia risk might be reduced and to identify the precise timing and nature of possible beneficial interventions.

REFERENCES

1. Reitz C, Brayne C, Mayeux R. Epidemiology of Alzheimer disease. Nat Rev Neurol 2011;7(3): 137–52.
2. Barnes DE, Yaffe K. The projected effect of risk factor reduction on Alzheimer's disease prevalence. Lancet Neurol 2011;10(9):819–28.
3. Bettens K, Sleegers K, Van Broeckhoven C. Current status on Alzheimer disease molecular genetics: from past, to present, to future. Hum Mol Genet 2010;19(R1):R4–11.
4. Saxena S, Caroni P. Selective neuronal vulnerability in neurodegenerative diseases: from stressor thresholds to degeneration. Neuron 2011;71(1):35–48.
5. Morris HR, Steele JC, Crook R, et al. Genome-wide analysis of the parkinsonism-dementia complex of Guam. Arch Neurol 2004;61(12):1889–97.
6. Whalley LJ, Dick FD, McNeill G. A life-course approach to the aetiology of late-onset dementias. Lancet Neurol 2006;5(1):87–96.
7. Zeki Al Hazzouri A, Haan MN, Kalbfleisch JD, et al. Life-course socioeconomic position and incidence of dementia and cognitive impairment without dementia in older Mexican Americans: results from the Sacramento area Latino study on aging. Am J Epidemiol 2011;173(10):1148–58.
8. Boyle PA, Wilson RS, Schneider JA, et al. Processing resources reduce the effect of Alzheimer pathology on other cognitive systems. Neurology 2008;70(17):1534–42.
9. Prince MJ, de Rodriguez JL, Noriega L, et al. The 10/66 Dementia Research Group's fully operationalised DSM-IV dementia computerized diagnostic algorithm, compared with the 10/66 dementia algorithm and a clinician diagnosis: a population validation study. BMC Public Health 2008;8:219.
10. Llibre Rodriguez JJ, Ferri CP, Acosta D, et al. Prevalence of dementia in Latin America, India, and China: a population-based cross-sectional survey. Lancet 2008;372(9637):464–74.
11. Ferri CP, Prince M. 10/66 Dementia Research Group: recently published survey data for seven Latin America sites. Int Psychogeriatr 2010;22(1): 158–9.
12. Fratiglioni L, Launer LJ, Andersen K, et al. Incidence of dementia and major subtypes in Europe: a collaborative study of population-based cohorts. Neurologic Diseases in the Elderly Research Group. Neurology 2000;54(11 Suppl 5):S10–5.
13. Lobo A, Launer LJ, Fratiglioni L, et al. Prevalence of dementia and major subtypes in Europe: a collaborative study of population-based cohorts. Neurologic Diseases in the Elderly Research Group. Neurology 2000;54(11 Suppl 5):S4–9.
14. Letenneur L, Launer LJ, Andersen K, et al. Education and the risk for Alzheimer's disease: sex makes a difference. EURODEM pooled analyses. EURODEM Incidence Research Group. Am J Epidemiol 2000;151(11):1064–71.
15. Jagger C, Andersen K, Breteler MM, et al. Prognosis with dementia in Europe: a collaborative study of population-based cohorts. Neurologic Diseases in the Elderly Research Group. Neurology 2000; 54(11 Suppl 5):S16–20.
16. Burns A, Robert P. The National Dementia Strategy in England. BMJ 2009;338:b931.
17. Wing JK, Nixon JM, Mann SA, et al. Reliability of the PSE (ninth edition) used in a population study. Psychol Med 1977;7(3):505–16.
18. Copeland JR, Kelleher MJ, Kellett JM, et al. A semistructured clinical interview for the assessment of diagnosis and mental state in the elderly: the Geriatric Mental State Schedule. I. Development and reliability. Psychol Med 1976;6(3):439–49.

19. Hachinski VC, Lassen NA, Marshall J. Multi-infarct dementia. A cause of mental deterioration in the elderly. Lancet 1974;2(7874):207–10.

20. Small GW, Rabins PV, Barry PP, et al. Diagnosis and treatment of Alzheimer disease and related disorders. Consensus statement of the American Association for Geriatric Psychiatry, the Alzheimer's Association, and the American Geriatrics Society. JAMA 1997;278(16):1363–71.

21. Ivan CS, Seshadri S, Beiser A, et al. Dementia after stroke: the Framingham Study. Stroke 2004;35(6): 1264–8.

22. Jack CR Jr, Albert MS, Knopman DS, et al. Introduction to the recommendations from the National Institute on Aging-Alzheimer's Association workgroups on diagnostic guidelines for Alzheimer's disease. Alzheimers Dement 2011;7(3):257–62.

23. Whalley LJ, Deary IJ, Appleton CL, et al. Cognitive reserve and the neurobiology of cognitive aging. Ageing Res Rev 2004;3(4):369–82.

24. ADAPT Research Group, Meinert CL, McCaffrey LD, et al. Alzheimer's Disease Anti-inflammatory Prevention Trial: design, methods, and baseline results. Alzheimers Dement 2009;5(2):93–104.

25. Hendrie HC, Hall KS, Ogunniyi A, et al. Alzheimer's disease, genes, and environment: the value of international studies. Can J Psychiatry 2004;49(2):92–9.

26. Hendrie HC, Murrell J, Gao S, et al. International studies in dementia with particular emphasis on populations of African origin. Alzheimer Dis Assoc Disord 2006;20(3 Suppl 2):S42–6.

27. Ogunniyi A, Hall KS, Gureje O, et al. Risk factors for incident Alzheimer's disease in African Americans and Yoruba. Metab Brain Dis 2006;21(2–3): 235–40.

28. Hall KS, Gao S, Unverzagt FW, et al. Low education and childhood rural residence: risk for Alzheimer's disease in African Americans. Neurology 2000;54(1): 95–9.

29. Evans RM, Emsley CL, Gao S, et al. Serum cholesterol, APOE genotype, and the risk of Alzheimer's disease: a population-based study of African Americans. Neurology 2000;54(1):240–2.

30. McGonigal G, Thomas B, McQuade C, et al. Epidemiology of Alzheimer's presenile dementia in Scotland, 1974-88. BMJ 1993;306(6879):680–3.

31. Whalley LJ, Thomas BM, McGonigal G, et al. Epidemiology of presenile Alzheimer's disease in Scotland (1974-88). I. Non-random geographical variation. Br J Psychiatry 1995;167(6):728–31.

32. Whalley LJ, Thomas BM, Starr JM. Epidemiology of presenile Alzheimer's disease in Scotland (1974-88). II. Exposures to possible risk factors. Br J Psychiatry 1995;167(6):732–8.

33. Whalley LJ. Early-onset Alzheimer's disease in Scotland: environmental and familial factors. Br J Psychiatry Suppl 2001;40:s53–9.

34. Starr JM, Thomas BM, Whalley LJ. Familial or sporadic clusters of presenile Alzheimer's disease in Scotland: II. Case kinship. Psychiatr Genet 1997; 7(4):147–52.

35. Starr JM, Thomas BM, Whalley LJ. Familial or sporadic clusters of presenile dementia in Scotland: I. Parental causes of death in Alzheimer and vascular presenile dementias. Psychiatr Genet 1997;7(4):141–6.

36. Schneider JA, Arvanitakis Z, Leurgans SE, et al. The neuropathology of probable Alzheimer disease and mild cognitive impairment. Ann Neurol 2009;66(2): 200–8.

37. Rocca WA, Petersen RC, Knopman DS, et al. Trends in the incidence and prevalence of Alzheimer's disease, dementia, and cognitive impairment in the United States. Alzheimers Dement 2011;7(1):80–93.

38. Hebert LE, Bienias JL, Aggarwal NT, et al. Change in risk of Alzheimer disease over time. Neurology 2010; 75:786–91.

39. Bienias JL, Beckett LA, Bennett DA, et al. Design of the Chicago Health and Aging Project (CHAP). J Alzheimers Dis 2003;5:349–55.

40. Hall KS, Ogunniyi AO, Hendrie HC, et al. A cross-cultural community based study of dementias: methods and performance of the survey instrument, Indianapolis, U.S.A., and Ibadan, Nigeria. Int J Methods Psychiatr Res 1996;6:129–42.

41. Juster FT, Suzman R. An overview of the Health and Retirement Study. J Hum Resour 1995;30:S7–56.

42. Ritchie K, Kildea D. Is senile dementia "age-related" or "ageing-related"?–evidence from meta-analysis of dementia prevalence in the oldest old. Lancet 1995; 346(8980):931–4.

43. MacDonald SW, DeCarlo CA, Dixon RA. Linking biological and cognitive aging: toward improving characterizations of developmental time. J Gerontol B Psychol Sci Soc Sci 2011;66(Suppl 1):i59–70.

44. Zekry D, Herrmann FR, Grandjean R, et al. Demented versus non-demented very old inpatients: the same comorbidities but poorer functional and nutritional status. Age Ageing 2008;37(1):83–9.

45. Sohal RS, Mockett RJ, Orr WC. Mechanisms of aging: an appraisal of the oxidative stress hypothesis. Free Radic Biol Med 2002;33(5):575–86.

46. Bartosz G. Non-enzymatic antioxidant capacity assays: limitations of use in biomedicine. Free Radic Res 2010;44(7):711–20.

47. Scarmeas N, Luchsinger JA, Mayeux R, et al. Mediterranean diet and Alzheimer disease mortality. Neurology 2007;69(11):1084–93.

48. Lloyd-Jones DM, Leip EP, Larson MG, et al. Prediction of lifetime risk for cardiovascular disease by risk factor burden at 50 years of age. Circulation 2006; 113(6):791–8.

49. Yaffe K, Kanaya A, Lindquist K, et al. The metabolic syndrome, inflammation, and risk of cognitive decline. JAMA 2004;292(18):2237–42.

50. Luchsinger JA, Tang MX, Shea S, et al. Plasma homocysteine levels and risk of Alzheimer disease. Neurology 2004;62(11):1972–6.

51. Zylberstein DE, Lissner L, Björkelund C, et al. Midlife homocysteine and late-life dementia in women. A prospective population study. Neurobiol Aging 2011;32(3):380–6.

52. Dangour AD, Whitehouse PJ, Rafferty K, et al. B-vitamins and fatty acids in the prevention and treatment of Alzheimer's disease and dementia: a systematic review. J Alzheimers Dis 2010;22(1):205–24.

53. Sinclair KD, Allegrucci C, Singh R, et al. DNA methylation, insulin resistance, and blood pressure in offspring determined by maternal periconceptional B vitamin and methionine status. Proc Natl Acad Sci U S A 2007;104(49):19351–6.

54. Ruxton CH, Reed SC, Simpson MJ, et al. The health benefits of omega-3 polyunsaturated fatty acids: a review of the evidence. J Hum Nutr Diet 2004; 17(5):449–59.

55. Dangour AD, Clemens F, Elbourne D, et al. A randomised controlled trial investigating the effect of n-3 long-chain polyunsaturated fatty acid supplementation on cognitive and retinal function in cognitively healthy older people: the Older People And n-3 Long-chain polyunsaturated fatty acids (OPAL) study protocol [ISRCTN72331636]. Nutr J 2006;5:20.

56. Glymour MM, Kosheleva A, Wadley VG, et al. Geographic distribution of dementia mortality: elevated mortality rates for black and white Americans by place of birth. Alzheimer Dis Assoc Disord 2011;25(3):196–202.

57. Helzner EP, Luchsinger JA, Scarmeas N, et al. Contribution of vascular risk factors to the progression in Alzheimer disease. Arch Neurol 2009;66(3): 343–8.

The Molecular Pathology of Alzheimer's Disease

Charles R. Harrington, PhD

KEYWORDS

- Alzheimer's disease • Tau protein • Amyloid-β protein
- Neurofibrillary tangles • Plaques
- Protein aggregation disorders

List of Key Learning Points

- The pathologic hallmarks of Alzheimer's disease are the presence of both neurofibrillary tangles and senile plaques, first described in a patient with presenile dementia by Alois Alzheimer.

- Neurofibrillary pathology consists of intraneuronal fibrils present in tangles, and in neurites found both throughout the neuropil and in neuritic senile plaques.

- Neurofibrillary pathology in Alzheimer's disease consists of paired helical filaments comprising tau protein.

- Amyloid pathology occurs as the deposition of amyloid-β (Aβ) protein within senile plaques and in the form of diffuse deposits throughout the neuropil. In addition, it can be found as deposits around blood vessels.

- Aβ deposits derive from the processing of a transmembrane-spanning Aβ protein precursor (APP) to release an extracellular Aβ peptide of 40 to 43 amino acids in length; larger peptides form more insoluble Aβ deposits.

- Mutations in APP and the presenilin proteins 1 and 2 cause familial Alzheimer's disease and result in increased deposition of insoluble Aβ. Presenilin 1 possesses the catalytic sites of a tetrameric γ-secretase complex that cleaves APP, with the aid of β-secretase, to Aβ peptides.

- Tau mutations cause tauopathy in conditions other than Alzheimer's disease in the absence of amyloid pathology. These conditions include frontotemporal dementia syndromes, and indicate that amyloid is not essential to cause dementia.

- Tau pathology in Alzheimer's disease precedes amyloid pathology by 2 decades.

- Molecular imaging of amyloid in Alzheimer's disease using Pittsburgh B compound and the future development of selective tau ligands indicate that knowledge of the pathogenesis of Alzheimer's disease will be greatly improved by direct visualization of the pathology in humans.

The German psychiatrist Alois Alzheimer presented the original description for a 55-year-old patient who had suffered with presenile dementia and who had the unique combination of both senile plaques and neurofibrillary degeneration in her brain.[1] Alzheimer was prompted to consider this case as representing a specific disease process in which the neurofibrillary pathology made it particularly distinctive. In just 2 pages, Alzheimer had described the pathologic basis for the

The author is Senior Research Fellow at University of Aberdeen and Chief Scientific Officer for TauRx Therapeutics Ltd, Singapore.
Division of Applied Health Sciences, School of Medicine and Dentistry, Institute of Medical Sciences, University of Aberdeen, Liberty Building, Foresterhill Road, Aberdeen AB25 2ZP, Scotland, UK
E-mail address: c.harrington@abdn.ac.uk

Neuroimag Clin N Am 22 (2012) 11–22
doi:10.1016/j.nic.2011.11.003

disease to be given his name. By 2010, more than 9000 articles related to Alzheimer's disease were published in a single year.

The pathologies that Alzheimer observed at autopsy can now be examined during life by molecular imaging techniques that allow an even greater insight into the pathogenesis of the disease and the means to assess therapeutic efficacy. This article focuses on the molecular pathology found in Alzheimer's disease, namely that of tau protein and amyloid-β (Aβ) protein (Fig. 1).

TAU PROTEIN PATHOLOGY IN ALZHEIMER'S DISEASE
Normal Tau Protein

Tau proteins are a family of microtubule-associated proteins. Tau proteins are predominantly expressed in neurons, where they play an important role in the assembly and stabilization of tubulin monomers into microtubules that constitute the neuronal cytoskeletal network. Microtubules are essential in morphogenesis, cell division, and intracellular trafficking of organelles. At physiologic concentrations tau proteins stabilize microtubules as tracks for intracellular transport, but in excess they interfere with transport down the axon. Tau also plays a role in signal transduction through its interaction with phospholipase C-γ, interacts with actin and the plasma membrane, is involved in anchoring of protein kinases and phosphatases, and is important in neurite outgrowth.[2]

Human tau protein in the central nervous system exists in 6 isoforms, ranging from 352 to 441 amino acids in length and derived by alternative mRNA splicing from a single gene (MAPT) located on

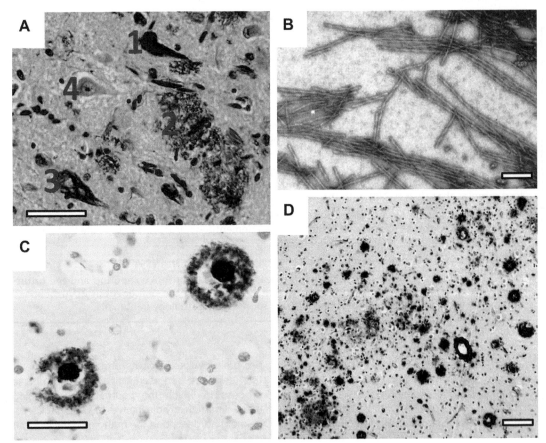

Fig. 1. Neuropathology of Alzheimer's disease is characterized by tau and amyloid-β (Aβ) pathologies. (A) Tau pathology involves intracellular accumulations of fibrous tau in neurofibrillary tangles within pyramidal neurons (1) and in the neurites of plaques (2), and throughout the neuropil. The NFTs eventually become extracellular ghost tangles (3) once the cytoplasmic membrane has burst. An unaffected neuron is also seen (4). (B) Paired helical filaments (PHFs) extracted from Alzheimer's disease brain tissue. (C, D) Aβ pathology in Alzheimer's disease showing plaques with cores (C); diffuse cortical amyloid staining and amyloid angiopathy surrounding a blood vessel (D). (A, C, D) Tau and amyloid pathology visualized using monoclonal anti-tau and polyclonal anti-Aβ; scale bars, 50 μm. (B) Electron microscopy of negative-stained PHF preparations; scale bar, 250 nm.

chromosome 17. The domains of tau protein are depicted in **Fig. 2**. There are 2 inserts in the acidic N-terminal domain encoded by exons 2 and 3. Each isoform contains either 3 or 4 tandem repeats of 31 or 32 amino acids located in the C-terminal portion of the molecule. The additional repeat is encoded by exon 10. These repeats are both rich in basic amino acids and capable of binding to an acidic domain of tubulin. Similar microtubule-binding repeats are found in the carboxy-terminal domain of high molecular weight microtubule-associated proteins (MAPs), such as MAP2. The different MAPs serve specific functions; tau is predominantly axonal in location, whereas MAP2 is restricted to the somatodendritic part of the neuron.

Neurofibrillary tangles (NFTs) are intraneuronal inclusions that form in a few susceptible types of neurons. NFTs are composed of aberrant tau protein polymers in the form of paired helical filaments (PHFs) (see **Fig. 1**B). There is considerable evidence in support of Alzheimer's view on the importance of neurofibrillary tangles in dementia. The neurofibrillary tau pathology is closely linked to intellectual status antemortem,[3–6] and deposition of diffuse amyloid can be extensive in intellectually normal elderly cases. By contrast, there are no reports of preservation of normal cognitive functioning in the presence of numerous neocortical tangles. The density of neuritic plaques, rather than amyloid deposits, tends to correlate better

both with the biochemical measure of PHF-tau and with cognitive dysfunction. Further studies also confirm that Aβ load does not predict neuronal loss, synapse loss, or dementia.[7,8] Furthermore, there is considerable overlap in the levels of Aβ deposition found in Alzheimer's disease and nondemented patients,[9] which is not the case with PHF accumulation.[10] The PHF-tau content in Alzheimer's disease tissue exceeds that found in control tissue by 19-fold, and the difference is even greater for brain regions such as temporal cortex.[10] The accumulation of PHFs is accompanied by a corresponding loss of normal soluble tau, in excess of the loss due to normal aging.[11] By contrast, the levels of Aβ in nearly half of the cases of Alzheimer's disease are found to overlap the levels found in controls, regardless of *APOE* genotype.[9] These findings argue against the hypothesis that Aβ deposition induces a direct toxic effect on neurons in the human brain, and rather poses the question as to exactly how tau and amyloid pathologies are connected.

Tau pathology is closely linked with synaptic loss, and Terry and colleagues[7] first reported that loss of synapses provided a better correlate of cognitive deficit than neurofibrillary tangles, a finding supported by others.[12,13] The tauopathy of Alzheimer's disease follows a characteristic pattern of spread of tau aggregation pathology, initially described by Braak and Braak (**Fig. 3**).[14] NFT pathology is most severe when it begins in

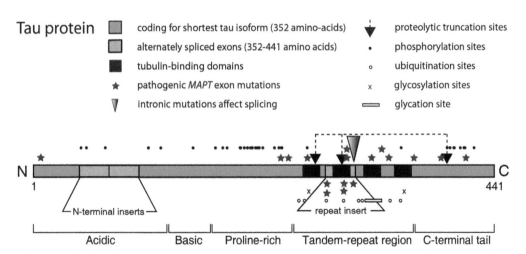

Fig. 2. Tau protein. Six isoforms of central nervous system tau are derived by alternative splicing of exons 2, 3, and 10 (*pink*), and the largest isoform is 441 amino acids in length. A tandem-repeat region in the C-terminal half of the molecule is involved in tubulin binding. Mutations that cause frontotemporal dementia and related disorders are associated with 2 major classes of mutation (*red stars*): (**1**) missense mutations that affect the assembly of microtubules and enhance the assembly of tau into filaments; (**2**) mutations surrounding the intron-exon boundaries that affect the splicing of exon 10, including intronic mutations that disrupt a predicted mRNA stem-loop structure and lead to an increased expression of exon 10. Sites of posttranslational modification of tau protein are indicated here and in the text.

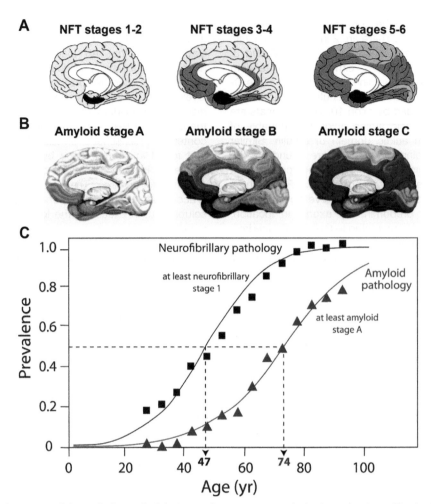

Fig. 3. Braak staging of the pathology of Alzheimer's disease. Neuropathologic evaluation of brains led to Braak staging based on immunohistochemical staining of tau pathology. (*A*) The sequence of spread of tangle pathology; the 6 neurofibrillary Braak stages have been combined to make 3 representative images. (*B*) By contrast, amyloid levels show relatively poor levels of staging. (*C*) Original data from 1997 show that tau pathology is initiated early, and precedes amyloid by at least 20 years. NFT, neurofibrillary tangle. ([*C*] *From* Duyckaerts C. Tau pathology in children and young adults: can you still be unconditionally baptist? Acta Neuropathol 2011;121:146; with permission; and [*A, B*] Braak H, Braak E. Frequency of stages of Alzheimer-related lesions in different age categories. Neurobiol Aging 1997;18:353, 354; with permission.)

the hippocampus and entorhinal cortex and, with progression, spreads to temporal, parietal, and frontal cortices. The process of tau aggregation begins in the neocortical regions well before NFTs appear.[15,16] Tau aggregation, in the form of proteolytically stable PHF-tau, is detected from Braak stage 2 onwards, whereas tangles that can be visualized by conventional microscopy do not appear until Braak stage 4 in the neocortex.

Duyckaerts[17] recently compared the temporal sequence of the appearance of tau and amyloid pathology from previously published Braak data[18] to show that tau pathology in the medial temporal lobe precedes Aβ accumulation by more than 2 decades (see **Fig. 3**). Furthermore, tau pathology is observed in a high proportion of children in the absence of Aβ accumulation.[19]

Mutations in the MAPT Gene that Cause Dementia

Mutations in the *MAPT* gene that cause neurodegenerative tauopathies other than Alzheimer's disease, namely progressive supranuclear palsy, argyrophilic grain disease, and a variety of frontotemporal disease syndromes, have been identified. At the ultrastructural level, the tau filaments in these patients consist mainly of straight or twisted-ribbon filaments rather than the PHFs typical of Alzheimer's disease.[20] Although mutations in the *MAPT* gene have not been found in Alzheimer's disease, the discovery that such mutations can cause dementia in the absence of β-amyloid pathology asserts that tau pathology need not be a secondary consequence of amyloid deposition.

There are 2 main classes of tau mutations: those that affect alternative splicing of the *MAPT* gene and those that directly affect the function of the protein. Mostly they cluster in the vicinity of the tandem-repeat domain of tau, as shown in **Fig. 2**. Mutations in the 5′-splice site of exon 10 destabilize the intron 10 stem-loop structure, which increases production of the 4-repeat isoforms.[21–24] Recombinant tau proteins carrying missense mutations or the deletion mutation (K280Δ) have a decreased ability to promote microtubule assembly, which is more marked for 3-repeat than for 4-repeat isoforms.[25–27] A decrease in the binding of tau to microtubules could destabilize them over time and disrupt axonal transport. The tau mutations could also lead to increases in free cytosolic tau and an increased propensity to form insoluble tau aggregates.[28] Of the mutations tested, the P301L and K280Δ mutations in exon 10 have the greatest effect on microtubule assembly. The P301L mutation has the greatest potential for fibril formation, and spherical structures are obtained by incubation of the mutant protein in the absence of heparin.[29] Furthermore, filaments are produced in the brains of mice that are transgenic for this mutant form of tau protein.[30] The mutations N279K and S305N, on the other hand, do not show any decreased ability to promote microtubule assembly. The latter mutations increase the splicing-in of exon 10. It is possible that subtle changes in the ratio between 4-repeat and 3-repeat tau isoforms may be sufficient to cause neurodegeneration over a prolonged period. Greater distances between the microtubules and fewer microtubules per process were observed with the V337M mutant isoform.[31] The varied ways by which the mutations affect the processing and function of tau are probably responsible for the phenotypic heterogeneity observed in patients with FTDP-17 (frontotemporal dementia with parkinsonism–17).[32–34]

Posttranslational Modifications of Tau Protein

The distinctive feature of Alzheimer's disease is the substantial redistribution of tau protein from its normal axonal location into somatodendritic PHFs,[10,35] the mechanism whereby this occurs being poorly understood. Tau protein is subject to several posttranslational modifications that may affect this distribution, including ubiquitination, phosphorylation, glycosylation, nonenzymatic glycation, and oxidation. Sites where these changes occur are depicted schematically in **Fig. 2**. Further changes that are observed in Alzheimer's disease are the proteolytic truncation of tau and its aggregation into oligomers and PHFs.

Expression of the different tau isoforms is developmentally regulated, and the extent of phosphorylation and glycosylation affects the function of the protein. A combination of kinase and phosphatase activity contributes to the extent of phosphorylation of tau, both in normal situations and in Alzheimer's disease.[2] Thus, tau from the neonate is phosphorylated at more sites than is tau from adult brain, and tau phosphorylation in developing brain is more dynamic than in adult brain. Phosphorylated tau is unable to bind microtubules, although the phosphorylation of tau has been found to be inhibitory for the aggregation of tau in vitro.[36,37]

O-Linked *N*-acetyl glucosamination is a dynamic and abundant posttranslational modification that can operate reciprocally with Ser-/Thr- phosphorylation.[38] Phosphorylation of Ser-/Thr- residues in PHF-tau would decrease the occurrence of *O*-GlcNAc in PHFs. Modification of PHF-tau, but not normal tau, by *N*-linked glycosylation has been reported.[39] By contrast, *N*-linked glycosylation usually occurs cotranslationally and is considered a less dynamic modification. Deglycosylation of PHFs, however, converts them into straight filaments, suggesting that *N*-linked glycosylation may contribute to the maintenance of the PHF structure.[39]

It is likely that ubiquitination, nonenzymatic glycation, and oxidation are late events that arise in older neurons as levels of oxidative stress increase with aging.[40] The first 2 of these changes are observed in the vicinity of the tandem-repeat region of tau, where the insoluble tangles are probably subject to futile attempts by the neuron to remove proteolytically resistant PHF-tau. By contrast, the role of phosphorylation at sites outside the repeat domain is more dynamic, affecting the numerous surface-exposed substrates for the abundant cytoplasmic kinases and phosphatases.

Aggregation of Tau Protein in Alzheimer's Disease

Normal tau protein possesses little physical structure: α-helical, β-sheet, and β-turns are absent.[41] Nevertheless, tau aggregation through the repeat domain confers proteolytic stability on a short segment of the molecule that corresponds closely to that isolated from the PHF core. This fragment has the intrinsic capacity to propagate tau capture.[42] Although extracellular matrix proteins (heparin) and acidic proteins (RNA) can promote tau aggregation in vitro,[43–45] facilitation of tau aggregation may be attributable to a general property of macromolecular substrates that bind tau nonspecifically.[46] The substrates that initiate tau aggregation in vivo remain to be identified. It is possible that stochastic conformational changes to tau molecules occur with aging to cause sporadic Alzheimer's disease. Alternatively, conformational changes might be induced through interaction with other macromolecules, and tau aggregation may be seeded by cross-linked dimers or preformed tau aggregates extracted from the brain.[47,48]

Several neurodegenerative diseases in which there is aberrant protein aggregation are characterized by protein misfolding. These disorders have been given terms conformational diseases[49] or prionoses.[50] The deposits consist of highly ordered fibrils having a cross-β-pleated structure. Despite the absence of homology in the primary structure of various precursor proteins, the amyloid structure is common for many different amyloid disorders.

Full-length tau does not aggregate in physiologic conditions,[51] and this does not change when the protein has been hyperphosphorylated in vitro.[52] Tau can be made to assemble into filaments in non-physiologic buffers and at high protein concentrations,[53] or when tau aggregation is facilitated by coincubation of tau protein with sulfated glycosaminoglycans.[43,45] Typically tau concentrations of between 40 and 100 µM are required, whereas direct measurements in the human brain indicate that tau protein concentrations are unlikely to exceed 1 µM within pyramidal cells.[37]

The tau protein present within the structural core of the PHF is a short fragment of nearly 100 amino acid residues in length, which derives from the repeat domain of tau.[54,55] This core-tau unit of the PHF has the remarkable property that it is able to reproduce itself at the expense of normal tau.[46] Normally, tau binds to tubulin monomers of the microtubule, as illustrated in **Fig. 4**. In Alzheimer's disease, however, tau accumulates as oligomers, which are subject to proteolysis, leaving a protease-resistant core. Such a core unit has the capacity to bind further tau molecules and initiate an autocatalytic process of tau aggregation.[42] Subsequently, oligomers assemble into the PHFs, as shown schematically in the lower panel of **Fig. 4**.

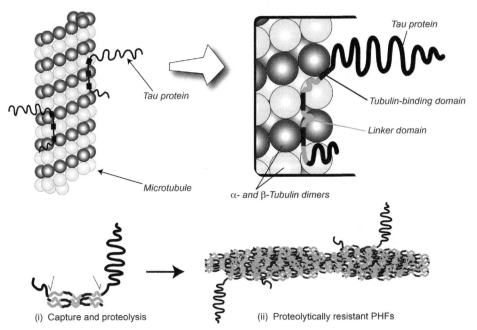

Fig. 4. Tau aggregation in Alzheimer's disease. Normal tau protein is active in the assembly and disassembly of microtubules comprising α-tubulin and β-tubulin subunits. Tau binds to these subunits through the tubulin-binding domain that is part of the tandem C-terminal repeats of tau. In the upper panel, the binding of a 3-repeat tau isoform to microtubules is shown. In Alzheimer's disease, tau aggregates through the repeat domain to form a resistant dimer or higher-order oligomer. The N- and C-termini are removed by endogenous proteolysis leaving oligomeric truncated tau, which acts as a seed for the nucleation of further tau capture and aggregation, before oligomers assemble into PHFs.

The capacity of tau protein pathology to propagate itself at the expense of normal tau has been confirmed in other studies. In an inducible tau transgenic model, tau pathology continued to progress even when expression of the tau transgene had been turned off.[56] Aggregated fibrils of a truncated tau fragment (residues 243–375) can be taken up into cells containing full-length tau and passed on to neighboring cells to seed aggregation.[57] Similarly, the transmission and spread of tau pathology from tau-mutant mice into normal mice was achieved whereby the latter mice were expressing human full-length tau protein.[58] These studies validate the proposal made by Braak and Braak[14] in 1991 that tau pathology spreads from the entorhinal cortex.

Once tau aggregation has been initiated, the only pathway available for clearance of the tau oligomers is the endosomal-lysosomal pathway, which becomes progressively congested with proteins from various sources, including Aβ. The capacity of neurons to clear proteolytically stable tau oligomers is therefore compromised, leading to uncontrolled progression of the tau aggregation process.[59]

In summary, therefore, Alzheimer's disease is characterized by altered neuronal metabolism of tau whereby the protein forms aggregates that then assemble into filaments having a defined paired helical structure. The appearance of oligomeric tau is correlated with cognitive deficit, and the progression of this process continues at an exponential rate, just as the prevalence of Alzheimer's disease increases in an age-dependent manner.

β-AMYLOID PATHOLOGY AND MOLECULAR GENETICS OF ALZHEIMER'S DISEASE

Mutations that cause Alzheimer's disease and influence Aβ protein deposition have been identified in 3 genes: Aβ protein precursor (APP) and 2 presenilin genes, PSNL1 and PSNL2. An updated list of these mutations can be found at http://www.alzforum.org. Further genetic risk factors, such as phosphatidylinositol-binding clathrin assembly protein (PICALM), are being identified through genome-wide association studies (GWAS).[60,61]

The Alzheimer's disease mutations of APP are either within or flanking the Aβ domain of APP, a domain that gives rise to the deposits of Aβ plaques throughout the cortex and, to a lesser extent, in the cerebellum.[62] APP exists in at least 5 isoforms, but its physiologic role in the brain is not understood. In the numbering of the largest APP isoform (770 residues), the 42-residue Aβ domain corresponds to residues 672 to 713 encoded for by exons 16 and 17 (Fig. 5). In one family,

a Swedish mutation results in the replacement of 2 amino acids (K670N and M671L), whereas other point mutations causing Alzheimer's disease include A692G, E693G, V715M, I716L, V717I, V717G, V717F, V717L, and L723P (see Fig. 5). Hereditary cerebral hemorrhage with amyloidosis—Dutch type, which exhibits severe congophilic angiopathy in the absence of plaques and tangles, is caused by the mutation E693Q.

APP is processed in different ways through the combined effect of several enzymes (see Fig. 5). First, the Aβ domain of APP can be cleaved within the middle by α-secretase in a nonamyloidogenic pathway. Second, there is an amyloidogenic pathway in which β-secretase[63] and γ-secretase[64] both cleave APP to create Aβ peptides. The β-secretase, also referred to as BACE (β-site APP cleaving enzyme), is located in the endoplasmic reticulum (ER) and Golgi. The γ-secretase acts as a transmembrane protease, generating Aβ of different lengths: $A\beta_{42}$ in pre-Golgi compartments, and $A\beta_{40}$ in later compartments and in the endocytic pathway. Subsequent growth of amyloid fibrils occurs by the assembly of seeds into protofibrils which, in turn, self-associate to form mature fibers.[65]

Some APP mutations result in overproduction of longer $A\beta_{42}$ forms that aggregate more readily than $A\beta_{40}$, and the ratio between Aβ peptides terminating at 40 residues and those with either 42 or 43 may have an effect on the acceleration of plaque formation.[66] The predominant form in diffuse and neuritic plaques tends to be the $A\beta_{42}$ residue form,[67] whereas the vascular deposits tend to be $A\beta_{40}$.[68]

Although the amyloid deposits in plaques are extracellular, degradation-resistant Aβ is also found within neurons, and this may be responsible for seeding the aggregation of other cellular proteins such as tau protein in Alzheimer's disease. The distribution of Aβ deposition, however, does not follow the same pattern as that of neurofibrillary degeneration (see Fig. 3).

The genes for the human presenilin proteins, PS1 and PS2, were identified in 1995,[69–71] and more than 170 mutations in PSNL1 and a further 13 in PSNL2 have been found to be causative for Alzheimer's disease (Fig. 6; for details on mutations, see http://www.molgen.ua.ac.be/ADMutations). Both are membrane-spanning proteins, which show extensive homology with each other and undergo proteolytic processing. Both proteins are normally localized in the nuclear envelope, the ER, and the Golgi, with PS2 being more predominant than the PS1 protein in the Golgi component. Just as mutations in APP lead to increases in the ratio of $A\beta_{42}$:$A\beta_{40}$, mutations in PS1 increase the levels of $A\beta_{42}$ in transfected cell lines,[72] transgenic

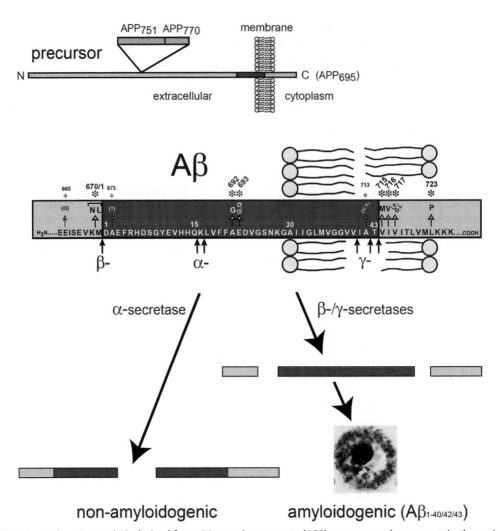

Fig. 5. Aβ protein. Aβ protein is derived from Aβ protein precursor (APP), a transmembrane protein that exists as various isoforms, the major form in neurons being 695 amino acids in length. The position of the major cleavage sites for α-secretase, β-secretase, and γ-secretase are shown in the more detailed lower panel, which gives the amino acid sequence for the Aβ domain. APP is subject to normal processing by α-secretase, a nonamyloidogenic pathway in which there is secretion of the N-terminal portion of the molecule. Aβ formation requires processing of APP by both β-secretase and γ-secretase. γ-Secretase (also known as BACE) is the rate-limiting enzyme of the two, and has been identified as a transmembrane aspartic protease. The pathogenic mutations, denoted by asterisks, are clustered around the β- and γ-secretase sites. The numbering of the mutations corresponds to the amino acid position in the largest APP isoform (APP770). Mutations not associated with disease are denoted by smaller letters and asterisks. The E693G mutation is associated with hereditary cerebral hemorrhage with amyloidosis (Dutch type).

mice,[73,74] and brain tissue from Alzheimer's disease patients carrying presenilin mutations.[75] Synthesized in the ER, PS1 undergoes a proteolytic maturation step when incorporated into the γ-secretase complex. This complex contains N-terminal and C-terminal fragments of PS1, and each of these fragments possesses the catalytic aspartyl residues embedded in transmembrane domains and required for the proteolytic activity on APP. The other

proteins in the tetrameric γ-secretase complex are nicastrin, anterior pharynx defective 1, and presenilin enhancer 2 (see **Fig. 6**), and details on their assembly and action have been reviewed recently.[76]

PS1 mutations facilitate apoptotic neuronal death in mice in the absence of amyloid formation, suggesting that PS1 need not necessarily exert its effect directly on amyloid deposition.[77] The accumulation of misfolded proteins in the lumen of

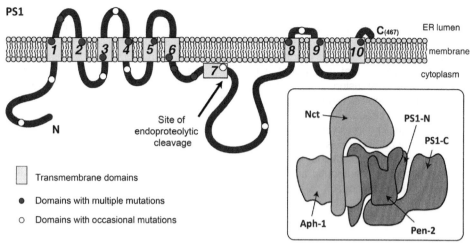

Fig. 6. Presenilin proteins and the γ-secretase complex. Both PS1 and PS2 are multiple transmembrane-spanning proteins showing considerable homology with each other. A model of PS1 indicates the putative topology of the protein, where 10 transmembrane or membrane-associated domains are indicated by yellow boxes. The location of clusters of mutations that cause early-onset Alzheimer's disease is indicated. These locations are predominantly in transmembrane domains or close to the cytoplasmic loop where protein is cleaved into N- and C-terminal fragments. ER, endoplasmic reticulum. The tetrameric γ-secretase (*inset*) consists of the resultant fragments (PS1-N and PS1-C), nicastrin (Nct), anterior pharynx defective 1 (Aph-1), and presenilin enhancer 2 (Pen-2).

the ER results in an unfolded-protein response, in which production of chaperones alleviates the increased demand on the existing protein-folding machinery. Altered chaperone levels, in turn, may influence the aggregation of other proteins.

Apolipoprotein E (apoE) is a plasma protein involved in cholesterol transport. Three major *APOE* alleles exist, namely ε2, ε3, and ε4, with ε3 being the most common. An association between the *APOE* ε4 allele and Alzheimer's disease was first demonstrated at Duke University,[78] and this finding has been replicated extensively. Possible biological explanations for the association of *APOE* genotype with Alzheimer's disease have included isoform-specific neurotoxic and/or neuroprotective effects of apoE and the binding of apoE to either Aβ or tau proteins in an isoform-dependent fashion.[78] Deposition and fibrillization of Aβ in transgenic mice is greatest in mice expressing the apoE4 isoform.[79]

A further link between Aβ and Alzheimer's disease comes from the recent identification that a yeast homologue of PICALM can modulate the toxicity of Aβ, suggesting that Aβ interferes with the ability of endocytosed transmembrane receptors, such as APP, to reach their proper destination.[80] It should be noted, however, that this connection has been made from studies in a yeast model and one in which tau protein is absent. Nevertheless, further studies are required on PICALM and other candidate proteins identified through GWAS.

CONNECTIONS BETWEEN AMYLOID AND TAU PATHOLOGY

Animal models of Alzheimer's disease are tools created to help better understand the relationship between the biochemical and pathologic changes in the brain and the impairment of memory and behavior. Rats and mice do not develop either amyloid or tau pathology, with or without normal aging. Aged dogs and nonhuman primates develop β-amyloidosis but not tau pathology,[81] while transgenic amyloid mice fail to exhibit abnormal tau fibrils.[82] Conversely, animal models of tau pathology fail to demonstrate amyloid pathology. Thus it is difficult to directly compare animal models with human Alzheimer's disease. Mice transgenic for both tau and amyloid have been created (see review[83] for examples), but it is difficult to replicate the pathologic levels of expression of both proteins, not to mention ensuring the regional selectivity of the two. Nevertheless, Ittner and Gotz[83] have proposed a "tau axis hypothesis" to link tau and Aβ pathology, based partly on the protection of dendrites from Aβ-induced toxicity being mediated by tau. Further testing of this hypothesis is required to establish that it plays a role in Alzheimer's disease.

FUTURE DIRECTIONS

Alzheimer's description of the pathologic findings of his patient in 1907, therefore, more than ever tells us that the human is the best model. There now exists the advantage that clinicians have the means to image this pathology during life at all stages of the disease process and to follow its progression. These advances establish that it is possible to image amyloid pathology using [^{11}C]Pittsburgh compound B (PIB),[84] or amyloid and tau pathology using [^{18}F]FDDNP.[85] Once tools for identifying tau-specific pathology are further developed, a better understanding of the pathogenesis of Alzheimer's disease may be reached. This advance will help in both the development of therapeutic agents and the assessment of their efficacy.

REFERENCES

1. Alzheimer A. Über eine eigenartige Erkrankung der Hirnrinde. Allg Z Psych Psych-gerich Med 1907; 64:146–8 [in German].
2. Buée L, Bussière T, Buée-Scherrer V, et al. Tau protein isoforms, phosphorylation and role in neuro-degenerative disorders. Brain Res Rev 2000;33: 95–130.
3. Giannakopoulos P, Hof PR, Michel JP, et al. Cerebral cortex pathology in aging and Alzheimer's disease: a quantitative survey of large hospital-based geriatric and psychiatric cohorts. Brain Res Rev 1997; 25:217–45.
4. Wilcock GK, Esiri MM. Plaques, tangles and dementia: a quantitative study. J Neurol Sci 1982; 56:407–17.
5. Duyckaerts C, Brion JP, Hauw JJ, et al. Quantitative assessment of the density of neurofibrillary tangles and senile plaques in senile dementia of the Alzheimer type. Comparison of immunocytochemistry with a specific antibody and Bodian's protargol method. Acta Neuropathol 1987;73:167–70.
6. Arriagada PW, Growdon JH, Hedley-White ET, et al. Neurofibrillary tangles but not senile plaques parallel duration and severity of Alzheimer's disease. Neurology 1992;42:631–9.
7. Terry RD, Masliah E, Salmon DP, et al. Physical basis of cognitive alterations in Alzheimer's disease: synapse loss is the major correlate of cognitive impairment. Ann Neurol 1991;30:572–80.
8. Gómez-Isla T, Hollister R, West H, et al. Neuronal loss correlates with but exceeds neurofibrillary tangles in Alzheimer's disease. Ann Neurol 1997;41:17–24.
9. Harrington CR, Louwagie J, Rossau R, et al. Influence of apolipoprotein E genotype on senile dementia of the Alzheimer and Lewy body types. Significance for etiological theories of Alzheimer's disease. Am J Pathol 1994;145:1472–84.
10. Mukaetova-Ladinska EB, Harrington CR, Roth M, et al. Biochemical and anatomical redistribution of tau protein in Alzheimer's disease. Am J Pathol 1993;143:565–78.

11. Mukaetova-Ladinska EB, Harrington CR, Roth M, et al. Alterations in tau protein metabolism during normal aging. Dementia 1996;7:95–103.
12. DeKosky ST, Scheff SW. Synapse loss in frontal cortex biopsies in Alzheimer's disease: correlation with cognitive severity. Ann Neurol 1990;27:457–64.
13. Price JL, Davis PB, Morris JC, et al. The distribution of tangles, plaques and related immunohistochemical markers in healthy aging and Alzheimer's disease. Neurobiol Aging 1991;12:295–312.
14. Braak H, Braak E. Neuropathological staging of Alzheimer-related changes. Acta Neuropathol 1991;82:239–59.
15. García-Sierra F, Wischik CM, Harrington CR, et al. Accumulation of C-terminally truncated tau protein associated with vulnerability of the perforant pathway in early stages of neurofibrillary pathology in Alzheimer's disease. J Chem Neuroanat 2001;22:65–77.
16. Mukaetova-Ladinska EB, Garcia-Sierra F, Hurt J, et al. Staging of cytoskeletal and β-amyloid changes in human isocortex reveals biphasic synaptic protein response during progression of Alzheimer's disease. Am J Pathol 2000;157:623–36.
17. Duyckaerts C. Tau pathology in children and young adults: can you still be unconditionally baptist? Acta Neuropathol 2011;121:145–7.
18. Braak H, Braak E. Frequency of stages of Alzheimer-related lesions in different age categories. Neurobiol Aging 1997;18:351–7.
19. Braak H, Del Tredici K. The pathological process underlying Alzheimer's disease in individuals under thirty. Acta Neuropathol 2011;121:171–81.
20. Spillantini MG, Goedert M. Tau protein pathology in neurodegenerative diseases. Trends Neurosci 1998; 21:428–33.
21. Hutton M, Lendon C, Rizzu P, et al. Association of missense and 5′-splice-site mutations in *tau* with the inherited dementia FTDP-17. Nature 1998;393: 702–5.
22. Spillantini MG, Murrell JL, Goedert M, et al. Mutation in the tau gene in familial multiple system tauopathy with presenile dementia. Proc Natl Acad Sci U S A 1998;95:7737–41.
23. Grover A, Houlden H, Baker M, et al. 5′ Splice site mutations in *tau* associated with the inherited dementia FTDP-17 affect a stem-loop structure that regulates alternative splicing of exon 10. J Biol Chem 1999;274:15134–43.
24. Varani L, Hasegawa M, Spillantini MG, et al. Structure of tau exon 10 splicing regulatory element RNA and destabilization by mutations of frontotemporal dementia and parkinsonism linked to chromosome 17. Proc Natl Acad Sci U S A 1999;96:8229–34.
25. Bugiani O, Murrell JR, Giaccone G, et al. Frontotemporal dementia and corticobasal degeneration in a family with a P301S mutation in *Tau*. J Neuropathol Exp Neurol 1999;58:667–77.

26. Rizzu P, van Swieten JC, Joose M, et al. High prevalence of mutations in the microtubule-associated protein tau in a population study of frontotemporal dementia in the Netherlands. Am J Hum Genet 1999;64:414–21.

27. Hasegawa M, Smith MJ, Goedert M. Tau proteins with FTDP-17 mutations have a reduced ability to promote microtubule assembly. FEBS Lett 1998; 437(3):207–10.

28. Hong M, Zhukareva V, Vogelsberg-Ragaglia V, et al. Mutation-specific functional impairments in distinct tau isoforms of hereditary FTDP-17. Science 1998; 282(5395):1914–7.

29. Nacharaju P, Lewis J, Easson C, et al. Accelerated filament formation from tau protein with specific FTDP-17 missense mutations. FEBS Lett 1999;447:195–9.

30. Lewis J, McGowan E, Rockwood J, et al. Neurofibrillary tangles, amyotrophy and progressive motor disturbance in mice expressing mutant (P301L) tau protein. Nature Genet 2000;25:402–5.

31. Frappier T, Liang NS, Brown K, et al. Abnormal microtubule packing in processes of SF9 cells expressing the FTDP-17 V337M tau mutation. FEBS Lett 1999;455:262–6.

32. Bird TD, Nochlin D, Poorkaj P, et al. A clinical pathological comparison of three families with frontotemporal dementia and identical mutations in the tau gene (P301L). Brain 1999;122:741–56.

33. D'Souza I, Poorkaj P, Hong M, et al. Missense and silent tau gene mutations cause frontotemporal dementia with parkinsonism-chromosome 17 type, by affecting multiple alternative RNA splicing regulatory elements. Proc Natl Acad Sci U S A 1999;96:5598–603.

34. Goedert M, Spillantini MG, Crowther RA, et al. Tau gene mutation in familial progressive subcortical gliosis. Nature Med 1999;5:454–7.

35. Harrington CR, Mukaetova-Ladinska EB, Hills R, et al. Measurement of distinct immunochemical presentations of tau protein in Alzheimer disease. Proc Natl Acad Sci U S A 1991;88:5842–6.

36. Schneider A, Biernat J, von Bergen M, et al. Phosphorylation that detaches tau protein from microtubules (Ser262, Ser214) also protects it against aggregation into Alzheimer paired helical filaments. Biochemistry 1999;38:3549–58.

37. Lai RY, Gertz HJ, Wischik DJ, et al. Examination of phosphorylated tau protein as a PHF-precursor at early stage Alzheimer's disease. Neurobiol Aging 1995;16:433–45.

38. Hayes BK, Hart GW. Novel forms of protein glycosylation. Curr Opinion Struct Biol 1994;4:692–6.

39. Wang JZ, Grundke-Iqbal I, Iqbal K. Glycosylation of microtubule-associated protein tau: an abnormal posttranslational modification in Alzheimer's disease. Nature Med 1996;2:871–5.

40. Stadtman ER. Protein oxidation and aging. Science 1992;257:1220–4.

41. Schweers O, Schönbrunn-Hanebeck E, Marx A, et al. Structural studies of tau protein and Alzheimer paired helical filaments show no evidence for β structure. J Biol Chem 1994;269:24290–7.

42. Wischik CM, Edwards PC, Lai RY, et al. Selective inhibition of Alzheimer disease-like tau aggregation by phenothiazines. Proc Natl Acad Sci U S A 1996;93:11213–8.

43. Pérez M, Valpuesta JM, Medina M, et al. Polymerization of τ into filaments in the presence of heparin: the minimal sequence required for τ-τ interaction. J Neurochem 1996;67:1183–90.

44. Kampers T, Friedhoff P, Biernat J, et al. RNA stimulates aggregation of microtubule-associated protein tau into Alzheimer-like paired helical filaments. FEBS Lett 1996;399:344–9.

45. Goedert M, Jakes R, Spillantini MG, et al. Assembly of microtubule-associated protein tau into Alzheimer-like filaments induced by sulphated glycosaminoglycans. Nature 1996;383:550–3.

46. Wischik CM, Lai RY, Harrington CR. Modelling prion-like processing of tau protein in Alzheimer's disease for pharmaceutical development. In: Avila J, Brandt R, Kosik KS, editors. Microtubule-associated proteins: modifications in disease. Amsterdam: Harwood Academic Publishers; 1997. p. 185–241.

47. Friedhoff P, von Bergen M, Mandelkow EM, et al. A nucleated assembly of Alzheimer paired helical filaments. Proc Natl Acad Sci U S A 1998;95:15712–7.

48. Yang LS, Ksiezak-Reding H. Ca^{2+} and Mg^{2+} selectively induces aggregates of PHF-tau but not normal human tau. J Neurosci Res 1999;55:36–43.

49. Carrell RW, Gooptu B. Conformational changes and disease—serpins, prions and Alzheimer's. Curr Opinion Struct Biol 1998;8:799–809.

50. Wisniewski T, Aucouuturier P, Soto C, et al. The prionoses and other conformational disorders. Amyloid. Int J Exp Clin Invest 1998;5:212–24.

51. Yanagawa H, Chung SH, Ogawa Y, et al. Protein anatomy: C-tail region of human tau protein as a crucial element in Alzheimer's paired helical filament formation in vitro. Biochemistry 1998;37:1979–88.

52. Crowther RA, Olesen OF, Smith MJ, et al. Assembly of Alzheimer-like filaments from full-length tau protein. FEBS Lett 1994;337:135–8.

53. Wille H, Drewes G, Biernat J, et al. Alzheimer-like paired helical filaments and antiparallel dimers formed from microtubule-associated protein tau in vitro. J Cell Biol 1992;118:573–84.

54. Wischik CM, Novak M, Thøgersen HC, et al. Isolation of a fragment of tau derived from the core of the paired helical filament of Alzheimer's disease. Proc Natl Acad Sci U S A 1988;85:4506–10.

55. Wischik CM, Novak M, Edwards PC, et al. Structural characterization of the core of the paired helical filament of Alzheimer disease. Proc Natl Acad Sci U S A 1988;85:4884–8.

56. SantaCruz K, Lewis J, Spires T, et al. Tau suppression in a neurodegenerative mouse model improves memory function. Science 2005;309:476–81.

57. Frost B, Jacks RL, Diamond MI. Propagation of tau misfolding from the outside to the inside of a cell. J Biol Chem 2009;284:12845–52.

58. Clavaguera F, Bolmont T, Crowther RA, et al. Transmission and spreading of tauopathy in transgenic mouse brain. Nature Cell Biol 2009;11:909–14.

59. Nixon RA, Cataldo AM, Mathews PM. The endosomal-lysosomal system of neurons in Alzheimer's disease pathogenesis: a review. Neurochem Res 2000;25:1161–72.

60. Harold D, Abraham R, Hollingworth P, et al. Genome-wide association study identifies variants at CLU and PICALM associated with Alzheimer's disease. Nature Genet 2009;41:1088–93.

61. Lambert JC, Heath S, Even G, et al. Genome-wide association study identifies variants at CLU and CR1 associated with Alzheimer's disease. Nature Genet 2009;41:1094–9.

62. Selkoe DJ. Cell biology of protein misfolding: The examples of Alzheimer's and Parkinson's diseases. Nature Cell Biol 2004;6:1054–61.

63. Vassar R, Bennett BD, Babu-Khan S, et al. β-Secretase cleavage of Alzheimer's amyloid precursor protein by the transmembrane aspartic protease BACE. Science 1999;286:735–41.

64. Wolfe MS, Xia W, Ostaszewski BL, et al. Two transmembrane aspartates in presenilin-1 required for presenilin endoproteolysis and γ-secretase activity. Nature 1999;398:513–7.

65. Harper JD, Lansbury PT Jr. Models of amyloid seeding in Alzheimer's disease and scrapie: mechanistic truths and physiological consequences of the time-dependent solubility of amyloid proteins. Ann Rev Biochem 1997;66:385–407.

66. Jarrett JT, Berger EP, Lansbury J, et al. The carboxy terminus of the β-amyloid protein is critical for the seeding of amyloid formation: implications for the pathogenesis of Alzheimer's disease. Biochemistry 1993;32:4693–7.

67. Iwatsubo T, Mann DM, Odaka A, et al. Amyloid β protein (Aβ) deposition: Aβ42(43) precedes Aβ40 in down syndrome. Ann Neurol 1995;37:294–9.

68. Suzuki N, Iwatsubo T, Odaka A, et al. High tissue content of soluble β1-40 is linked to cerebral amyloid angiopathy. Am J Pathol 1994;145:452–60.

69. Sherrington R, Rogaev EI, Liang Y, et al. Cloning of a gene bearing missense mutations in early-onset familial Alzheimer's disease. Nature 1995;375:754–60.

70. Rogaev EI, Sherrington R, Rogaeva EA, et al. Familial Alzheimer's disease in kindreds with missense mutations in a gene on chromosome 1 related to the Alzheimer's disease type 3 gene. Nature 1995;376:775–8.

71. Levy-Lahad E, Wasco W, Poorkaj P, et al. Candidate gene for the chromosome 1 familial Alzheimer's disease locus. Science 1995;269:973–7.

72. Citron M, Diehl TS, Gordon G, et al. Evidence that the 42- and 40-amino acid forms of amyloid β protein are generated from the β-amyloid precursor protein by different protease activities. Proc Natl Acad Sci USA 1996;93:13170–5.

73. Duff K, Eckman C, Zehr C, et al. Increased amyloid-β42(43) in brains of mice expressing mutant presenilin 1. Nature 1996;383:710–3.

74. Borchelt DR, Thinakaran G, Eckman CB, et al. Familial Alzheimer's disease-linked presenilin 1 variants elevate Aβ1-42/1-40 ratio in vitro and in vivo. Neuron 1996;17:1005–13.

75. Lemere CA, Lopera F, Kosik KS, et al. The E280A presenilin 1 Alzheimer mutation produces increased Aβ42 deposition and severe cerebellar pathology. Nature Med 1996;2:1146–50.

76. De Strooper B, Annaert W. Novel research horizons for presenilins and γ-secretases in cell biology and disease. Annu Rev Cell Dev Biol 2010;26:235–60.

77. Chui DH, Tanahashi H, Ozawa K, et al. Transgenic mice with Alzheimer presenilin 1 mutations show accelerated neurodegeneration without amyloid plaque formation. Nature Med 1999;5:560–4.

78. Strittmatter WJ, Saunders AM, Schmechel D, et al. Apolipoprotein E: high avidity binding to β-amyloid and increased frequency of type 4 allele in late-onset familial Alzheimer disease. Proc Natl Acad Sci USA 1993;90:1977–81.

79. Bales KR, Verina T, Cummins DJ, et al. Apolipoprotein E is essential for amyloid deposition in the APP^V717F transgenic mouse model of Alzheimer's disease. Proc Natl Acad Sci U S A 1999;96:15233–8.

80. Treusch S, Hamamichi S, Goodman JL, et al. Functional links between Aβ toxicity, endocytic trafficking, and Alzheimer's disease risk factors in yeast. Science 2011;334:1241–5.

81. Walker LC. Animal models of cerebral β-amyloid angiopathy. Brain Res Rev 1997;25:70–84.

82. Janus C, Chishti MA, Westaway D. Transgenic mouse models of Alzheimer's disease. Biochim Biophys Acta 2000;1502:63–75.

83. Ittner LM, Gotz J. Amyloid-β and tau—a toxic pas de deux in Alzheimer's disease. Nat Rev Neurosci 2011;12(2):67–72.

84. Klunk WE, Engler H, Nordberg A, et al. Imaging brain amyloid in Alzheimer's disease with Pittsburgh Compound-B. Ann Neurol 2004;55:306–19.

85. Shoghi-Jadid K, Small GW, Agdeppa ED, et al. Localization of neurofibrillary tangles and beta-amyloid plaques in the brains of living patients with Alzheimer disease. Am J Geriat Psychiatry 2002;10:24–35.

Clinical and Research Diagnostic Criteria for Alzheimer's Disease

Marie Sarazin, MD, PhD[a,b,c,d,e,*],
Leonardo Cruz de Souza, MD, PhD[a,b,c,d,e],
Stéphane Lehéricy, MD, PhD[a,b,c,d,f], Bruno Dubois, MD[a,b,c,d,e]

KEYWORDS

- Alzheimer • MCI • New criteria • Biomarkers
- Memory testing

NEW CONCEPTS FOR THE CLINICAL DEFINITION OF ALZHEIMER'S DISEASE

For more than 25 years, the diagnosis of Alzheimer's disease (AD) has been based on the National Institute of Neurological and Communicative Disorders and Stroke (NINCDS) and the Alzheimer's Disease and Related Disorders Association (ADRDA) criteria, according to which the diagnosis is classified as definite (clinical diagnosis with histologic confirmation), probable (typical clinical syndrome without histologic confirmation), or possible (atypical clinical features but no alternative diagnosis apparent; no histologic confirmation).[1] According to this definition, clinicians used the term AD to refer to a clinical dementia entity that typically presents with a characteristic progressive amnestic disorder with the subsequent appearance of other cognitive and neuropsychiatric changes that impair social function and activities of daily living.[2] In the NINCDS-ADRDA criteria, biological investigation (blood and cerebrospinal fluid [CSF]) and neuroimaging examination (computed tomography [CT] scan or magnetic resonance [MR] imaging) were only proposed to exclude other causes of the dementia syndrome (eg, vascular lesions, tumors, infectious or inflammatory processes). Typical sensitivity and specificity values for the diagnosis of probable AD with the use of NINCDS-ADRDA criteria are 81% and 73%, respectively.[3]

The recent advances in biomarkers of AD, which provide in vivo information about the pathophysiologic process associated with AD, have stimulated the proposal of new diagnostic criteria by the International Working Group (IWG) for New Research Criteria for the Diagnosis of AD.[4,5] According to this framework, the diagnosis of AD was reconceptualized as a clinical-biological entity with a specific clinical phenotype and confirmatory in vivo pathophysiologic evidence of AD. This combined clinical and biological approach may improve the accuracy of the diagnosis.[6–8] Because this new diagnostic framework no longer refers to dementia, it permits a clinical diagnosis to be established at an early prodromal/predementia stage of the disease that

a Université Pierre et Marie Curie Paris 6, Centre de Recherche de l'Institut du Cerveau et de la Moelle Epinière, UMR-S975, 47-83 Boulevard de l'Hôpital, 75013 Paris, France
b Inserm, U975, 47-83 Boulevard de l'Hôpital, 75013 Paris, France
c CNRS, UMR 7225, 47-83 Boulevard de l'Hôpital, 75013 Paris, France
d Institut du Cerveau et de la Moelle Epinière, ICM, 47-83 Boulevard de l'Hôpital, 75013 Paris, France
e Alzheimer Institute, Research and Resource Memory Centre, Centre de Référence des Démences Rares, Centre de Référence maladie d'Alzheimer jeune, AP-HP, Pitié-Salpêtrière Hospital, 47-83 Boulevard de l'Hôpital, 75013 Paris, France
f Centre de Neuroimagerie de Recherche–CENIR and Department of Neuroradiology, Pitié-Salpêtrière Hospital, 47-83 Boulevard de l'Hôpital, 75013 Paris, France
* Corresponding author. Alzheimer Institute, Research and Resource Memory Centre, Centre de Référence des Démences Rares, Centre de Référence maladie d'Alzheimer jeune, AP-HP, Pitié-Salpêtrière Hospital, 47-83 Boulevard de l'Hôpital, 75013 Paris, France.
E-mail address: marie.sarazin@psl.aphp.fr

Neuroimag Clin N Am 22 (2012) 23–32
doi:10.1016/j.nic.2011.11.004

was previously incorporated in the heterogeneous concept of mild cognitive impairment (MCI).

More recently, the National Institute of Aging-Alzheimer's Association (NIA-AA) workgroups published new diagnostic guidelines for AD[9–12] that also incorporate biological and imaging markers to establish an earlier diagnosis of AD.

In both diagnostic criteria,[4,13] a consideration of preclinical stages of AD is proposed, according to which the pathophysiologic process of the disease precedes the clinical manifestations. Because this condition has been studied, but there are no clinical implications at this time, this aspect of AD is not discussed in this article.

IDENTIFICATION OF THE CLINICAL SYMPTOMS OF AD AT AN EARLY STAGE
Progression of Cognitive Symptoms Follows the Progression of the Underlying Cerebral Lesions

The most prominent feature of AD is a decline in cognitive function.[2] In the early stages of AD, critical areas for episodic memory are already affected by neuropathologic changes (neurofibrillary degeneration) in medial temporal regions (hippocampal formations, parahippocampal gyrus, and entorhinal cortex). As a consequence, episodic memory deficit is an initial and reliable neuropsychological marker of AD.[14,15] Memory impairment of recent

events, unusual repeated omissions, and difficulty in learning new information characterize the first clinical signs. As the disease progresses, the clinical symptoms may involve language disorders, visuospatial and recognition deficits, and difficulties in executing more complex tasks of daily living, leading to dementia.[2] The progression of cognitive deficits is consistent with the extension of underlying pathologic lesions (more specifically, of tau lesions) through the neocortical associative areas, as established by Braak and Braak.[14]

Amnesic Syndrome of the Medial Temporal Type as a Marker of Hippocampal Damage

A limit for establishing an early AD diagnosis concerns the ability to identify the specific pattern of memory disorders in relation to damage to the hippocampal formations that characterize the disease and to distinguish them from age-related attention disorders, or from retrieval deficits that are seen in depression, frontal lobe dysfunction, subcortical dementia, or some vascular dementias. The neuropsychological testing, when adequate memory tests are used, can quantify and qualify the memory deficit and can therefore distinguish genuine memory impairment (eg, failure of information storage and new memory formation) from attention or retrieval disorders (such as normal aging or frontal disorders) (**Fig. 1**). More

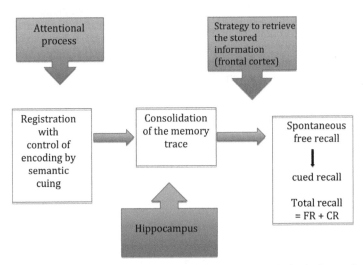

Fig. 1. Principle of examination of verbal episodic memory. The neuropsychological paradigm of the Free and Cued Selective Reminding Test (FCSRT) is based on the 3 different components of episodic memory: registration (by ensuring that all the items have been registered), storage, and retrieval. Verbal episodic memory is assessed by the spontaneous recall of items after delay, and the cued recall, by providing the semantic cues for facilitating access to stored information. Total recall, which is the sum of the spontaneous and the cued recalls, reflects the amount of information that is stored by the patient. A low total recall (ie, low free recall with an inefficiency of cueing [<71%]) suggests a deficit in storage caused by hippocampus damage, whereas a low free recall normalized by cueing (normal total recall) suggests a deficit in retrieval strategy caused by subcortical-frontal dysfunction. CR, cued recall; FR, free recall.

particularly, test paradigms that provide encoding specificity are of great interest and improve the diagnostic accuracy.[5] Within such memory paradigms, test materials are encoded along with specific cues (eg, semantic cues) that are used to control for an effective encoding and are subsequently presented to maximize retrieval. Memory tests that coordinate encoding and retrieval processes include the Free and Cued Selective Reminding Test (FCSRT) or similar cued recall paradigms.[16,17] The FCSRT can identify the amnesic syndrome of the medial temporal type (also called the hippocampal type) observed in AD, defined by (1) poor free recall (as in any memory disorders) and (2) decreased total recall caused by an insufficient effect of cueing. The low performance of total recall despite retrieval facilitation indicates poor storage of information. Measures of sensitivity to semantic cueing can successfully differentiate patients with AD from healthy controls, even when patients are matched to controls on their Mini-Mental State Examination (MMSE) scores or when disease severity is mild.[16,18,19] By isolating patients with an amnesic syndrome of the hippocampal type among those with MCI, the FCSRT is able to distinguish patients at an early stage of AD from MCI nonconverters with high sensitivity (80%) and specificity (90%).[19]

In an AD population, a recent MR imaging study showed that the performance of the FCSRT was correlated with the left medial temporal lobe volume assessed both by voxel-based morphometry analysis and the automatic volumetric method, reinforcing the idea that the measure of episodic memory by this test may be considered a useful clinical marker of medial temporal damage.[20] These correlations within the hippocampus were specially localized in the CA1 field, a region known to be involved in memory storage,[21] and to be affected early by AD neurobiological processes.[22]

The amnestic syndrome of the medial temporal type differs from functional and subcorticofrontal memory disorders, which are characterized by a low free recall performance with a normalization (or a quasinormalization) of the performance in total recall because of good efficacy of cueing.[23] This subcortical-frontal profile of memory impairment is observed in depression,[24] vascular dementia,[25] frontotemporal dementia,[26] and subcortical dementia,[23] showing its additional value for differential diagnosis.

Neuropsychological tests should also assess other cognitive functions that may be affected even at a mild stage of the disease, such as executive functions, visuospatial capacities, language, or semantic knowledge.

Severity of Disease

Different stages of severity are described in AD, from mild to moderate and severe dementia. In the recent AD criteria,[4,5,9] the terms prodromal AD, predementia AD, or AD at the stage of MCI (MCI caused by AD) were proposed in reference to the early stage of the disease.

The MMSE assesses global cognitive efficiency and it is generally used to evaluate dementia severity. Although MMSE is not a specific neuropsychological test for AD diagnosis, it is easy and quick to administer and can track the overall progression of cognitive decline. Longitudinal studies have shown that the mean annual rate of progression of cognitive impairment using MMSE is approximately 2 to 6 points. The Clinical Dementia Rating Scale (CDR), based on an overall evaluation of the patient's condition, offers incremental stages of severity.[27] Functional decline increases with disease progression. In the MCI stage, the patient can live alone. In mild stages of AD, patients require limited home care. In moderate stages, patients need supervision and regular assistance in most activities. In severe stages, residential health care may be required.

BIOMARKERS OF AD

The term biomarkers refers to "an objective measure of a biological or pathogenic process that can be used to evaluate disease risk or prognosis, to guide clinical diagnosis or to monitor therapeutic interventions."[28] These biomarkers include both neuroimaging and biological tools.

Structural Imaging Based on MR Imaging: Atrophy of Medial Temporal Structures as a Topographic and Neurodegenerative Marker

For many years, the use of CT and MR imaging in the evaluation of AD has been proposed for excluding neurosurgical lesions, such as brain tumors or subdural hematomas, or cerebrovascular lesions (cerebral infarcts, white matter lesions, microbleeds) that may account for vascular dementia. Modern neuroimaging extends beyond this traditional role of excluding other conditions and MR imaging is now considered an essential part of AD diagnosis.

The volume of the hippocampus is significantly reduced in AD compared with age-matched control subjects, by 30% to 40% in moderate AD, 15% to 30% in mild AD (MMSE >20), and about 10% to 12% in early AD (MMSE about 27).[29,30] Atrophy of medial temporal structures detected by high-resolution MR imaging is considered to be a reliable diagnostic marker at the

MCI stage,[29,30] and supports the diagnosis of AD.[5] A recent meta-analysis estimated that medial temporal atrophy has 73% sensitivity and 81% specificity for predicting whether patients with amnestic MCI will convert to dementia.[31] In the more advanced stage of AD, atrophy in temporal, parietal, and frontal neocortices is associated with language, praxic, visuospatial, and behavioral impairments.[32]

Cortical atrophy, especially hippocampal atrophy, assessed by MR imaging is considered a topographic biomarker.[4,29] Neuropathologic studies in patients with AD showed that the hippocampal volume measured in vivo by MR imaging correlates with tau deposition, Braak stage, and neuronal counts.[33] Moreover, atrophy of medial temporal structures was correlated with memory deficit.[20]

However, medial temporal atrophy is not specific enough to serve as an absolute criterion for the clinical diagnosis of AD at the MCI stage.[29] A decreased volume of the hippocampus can be observed in neurodegenerative conditions other than AD, even in depression and normal aging. The overlap of hippocampal volume measures between AD and normal aging limits its interpretation when considered without clinical data.

To facilitate clinical investigation, several rating scales have been developed to quantify the degree of medial temporal lobe atrophy by visual inspection of coronal T1-weighted MR imaging. Visual rating scales provide 80% to 85% sensitivity and specificity to distinguish patients with AD from those with no cognitive impairment.[34,35] These scales are widely used and can predict the risk of conversion to dementia in the MCI population.[34,35] New automated methods of segmentation are also valuable tools for measuring hippocampal volume[36,37] and may be useful in clinical practice in the future.

The combination of other markers (such as CSF biomarkers) with measures of hippocampal volume increases the accuracy of a diagnosis of early AD. However, rates of change in several structural measures, including whole brain, entorhinal cortex, hippocampal, and temporal lobe volumes, as well as ventricular enlargement, correlate closely with changes in cognitive performance, supporting their validity as markers of disease progression.[29]

Single-Photon Emission CT and Fluorodeoxyglucose Positron Emission Tomography as a Marker of Neuronal Dysfunction

Functional neuroimaging techniques include measurement of blood flow (^{99m}Tc-hexamethyl-propyleneamine oxime [HMPAO] or ^{133}Xe) with single-photon emission CT (SPECT), and positron emission tomography (PET).

SPECT has the advantage of greater availability than PET imaging but PET provides images with higher resolution. ^{99m}Tc-HMPAO SPECT is a useful neuroimaging technique for distinguishing AD from frontotemporal dementia (FTD) but a systematic review reported a clinical accuracy for patients with AD versus control individuals of only 74%.[38] However, recent work in a group with amnestic MCI showed that an automated quantitative tool for brain perfusion SPECT images using the mean activity in right and left parietal cortex and hippocampus was able to distinguish patients at an early stage of AD from patients with stable MCI (sensitivity, specificity, and accuracy of 82%, 90%, and 89%, respectively).[39]

PET with fluorodeoxyglucose (FDG) to measure glucose metabolism has shown good accuracy in distinguishing patients with AD, even at an early stage, from both normal control individuals and patients with non-AD dementias. This imaging method has been approved in the United States for diagnostic purposes. A meta-analysis has reported a sensitivity and specificity of 86% for the diagnosis of AD, although there were wide variations between studies.[40] A reduction of glucose metabolism in bilateral temporal parietal regions and in the posterior cingulate cortex is the most common finding in AD.[5,9,12]

CSF Amyloid and Tau Levels as Pathophysiologic Markers

The challenges for establishing an early diagnosis and for the development of disease-modifying drugs have created a need for biomarkers that reflect core pathologic elements of the disease.[28] The 2 core pathologic hallmarks of AD are (1) amyloid plaques, mainly composed of a heart of aggregated β-amyloid (Abeta) protein; and (2) neurofibrillary tangles (NFT), composed of abnormally hyperphosphorylated forms of the tau protein. In AD, the biomarkers that have been developed reflect amyloid and neurofibrillary tangle abnormalities. Because CSF is in direct contact with the extracellular space of the brain, the CSF is the optimal source of biological physiopathologic biomarkers.[28] The CSF levels of total tau (T-tau), phosphorylated tau (P-tau), and β-amyloid peptide 1-42 (Ab) can distinguish controls from individuals with AD, with a sensitivity and specificity between 80% and 90% even in the early stages of the disease.[28] In autopsy-proven AD, the P-tau/Ab ratio has the best sensitivity (91.6%) and specificity (85.7%) for differentiating AD from normal aging.[41] The combination of low Ab and high levels of T-tau and P-tau, or, more specifically, the abnormal ratio of Ab to P-Tau, are associated with high rates of progression from amnestic MCI to AD

dementia with a sensitivity of 95% and a specificity of 87%.[42]

Neuropathologic studies that analyzed correlations between the levels of in vivo CSF biomarkers

---

Box 1

Research criteria for the diagnosis of AD: revising the NINCDS-ADRDA criteria

Probable AD: A plus 1 or more supportive features (B, C, D, or E)

Core diagnostic criteria

A. Presence of an early and significant episodic memory impairment that includes the following features:

    1. Gradual and progressive change in memory function reported by patients or informants for more than 6 months

    2. Objective evidence of significantly impaired episodic memory on testing: this generally consists of recall deficit that does not improve significantly or does not normalize with cueing or recognition testing and after effective encoding of information has been controlled

    3. The episodic memory impairment can be isolated or associated with other cognitive changes at the onset of AD or as AD advances

Supportive features

B. Presence of medial temporal lobe atrophy: volume loss of hippocampi, entorhinal cortex, amygdala shown on MR imaging with qualitative ratings using visual scoring (referenced to well-characterized population with age norms) or quantitative volumetry of regions of interest (referenced to well-characterized population with age norms)

C. Abnormal CSF biomarker: low amyloid β1-42 concentrations, increased total tau concentrations, or increased phosphorylated tau concentrations, or combinations of the 3 (or other well-validated markers that have yet to be discovered)

D. Specific pattern on functional neuroimaging with PET

    Reduced glucose metabolism in bilateral temporal parietal regions

    Other well-validated ligands, including those that are expected to emerge, such as PiB or fluoroethyl-methylamino-2-naphthylethylidenemalononitrile

E. Proven AD autosomal dominant mutation within the immediate family

Exclusion criteria

History

    Sudden onset

    Early occurrence of the following symptoms: gait disturbances, seizures, behavioral changes

Clinical features

    Focal neurologic features including hemiparesis, sensory loss, visual field deficits

    Early extrapyramidal signs

Other medical disorders severe enough to account for memory and related symptoms

    Non-AD dementia

    Major depression

    Cerebrovascular disease

    Toxic and metabolic abnormalities, all of which may require specific investigations

    MR imaging fluid-attenuated inversion recovery or T2 signal abnormalities in the medial temporal lobe that are consistent with infectious or vascular insults

From Dubois B, Feldman HH, Jacova C, et al. Research criteria for the diagnosis of Alzheimer's disease: revising the NINCDS-ADRDA criteria. Lancet Neurol 2007;6:738; with permission.

with the intensity of the postmortem cerebral lesions found correlations between CSF Ab with amyloid plaque load and between CSF T-tau and P-tau with neurofibrillary tangles.[41,43] In a recent work using the new IWG criteria,[4,5] high CSF T-tau and P-tau, but not CSF Ab, were correlated with hippocampal atrophy, suggesting that CSF tau markers are related to the neuronal loss associated with AD.[44]

The combined analysis of the CSF biomarkers, specially the ratio P-tau/Ab, is also helpful for the differential diagnosis between AD and frontotemporal lobar degeneration (FTLD), whatever its behavioral presentation (FTD) or semantic dementia.[45] CSF biomarkers are able to distinguish FTLD with a sensitivity and specificity of around 90%. These results are similar to those from a previous study of patients with FTD shown at autopsy or by genetic studies.[46]

Pittsburgh Compound B PET Imaging as a Pathophysiologic Marker of Brain Amyloid Deposition

Amyloid imaging with PET represents a major advance in AD diagnosis, by enabling the detection and quantification of pathologic protein aggregations in the brain. Pittsburgh compound B labeled with carbon 11 (^{11}C-PiB), an analogue of the amyloid-binding thioflavin-T, is the most extensively studied and best validated tracer. ^{11}C-PiB binds specifically to fibrillar β-amyloid (Aβ) deposits, amyloid plaques, and vascular amyloid, but not appreciably to other protein aggregates such as NFTs or Lewy bodies.[47] ^{11}C-PiB binds nonspecifically to white matter, likely because of delayed clearance of the lipophilic compound from white matter.[48] Using clinical diagnosis as the gold standard, the sensitivity of ^{11}C-PiB for AD diagnosis has been reported as

80% to 100%, with most studies reporting sensitivities of 90% or greater.[49,50]

In most patients, the distribution of tracer uptake is diffuse and symmetric. The highest tracer uptake is consistently found in the prefrontal cortex, precuneus, and posterior cingulate cortex, closely followed by lateral parietal and temporal cortex and striatum, with lower tracer uptake in occipital cortex, globus pallidus, and thalamus.[50,51] ^{11}C-PiB-PET can identify patients with MCI who have amyloid deposition and who may be considered to be at an early clinical phase of AD. Longitudinal studies showed that patients with MCI with significant ^{11}C-PiB retention are at higher risk of developing AD dementia, in contrast with patients with MCI without significant ^{11}C-PiB retention.[52,53] ^{11}C-PiB-PET may be useful to distinguish cognitive deficit caused by AD from non-AD cognitive deficit.

PET imaging with ^{11}C-PiB may be useful in identifying atypical forms of AD, presenting either as a logopenic primary progressive aphasia[54] or a posterior cortical atrophy.[55,56] ^{11}C-PiB can also detect amyloid deposition in other dementia syndromes associated with β-amyloidosis to varying degrees, including cerebral amyloid angiopathy,[51] or Lewy body dementia (LBD).[57] In addition, amyloid PET imaging can improve the differential diagnosis of AD from FTD.[58] The significance of a negative ^{11}C-PiB scan in a patient clinically diagnosed with AD is not yet clear, but it may be explained by ^{11}C-PiB binding that it is insufficient for in vivo detection.[51]

INCORPORATING NEW TOOLS FOR THE DIAGNOSIS OF AD: THE NEW AD CRITERIA

In contrast with the previous AD diagnostic criteria published in 1984, the new IWG criteria[4,5]

Table 1
Categorization of AD biomarkers

	NIA-AA Recommendations (2011)		IWG Criteria (2007, 2010)	
	Biomarkers of Ab Deposition	Biomarkers of Neuronal Injury	Pathophysiologic Markers	Topographic Markers
CSF Ab42	Yes	No	Yes	No
CSF tau/P-tau	—	Yes	Yes	No
PET amyloid imaging	Yes	—	Yes	No
HV or MTLA by MR imaging	No	Yes	No	Yes
Rate of brain atrophy	No	Yes	No	Yes
FDG-PET	No	Yes	No	Yes
SPECT perfusion imaging	No	Yes	No	Yes

Abbreviations: HV, hippocampal volume; MTLA, medial temporal lobe atrophy.

incorporated biomarkers of the underlying pathophysiologic process in the diagnostic framework. The combination of clinical and biological approaches allows the establishment of a clinical diagnosis of AD without having to wait until a dementia syndrome develops. In this view, AD does not overlap with the concept of dementia. AD is considered to be a progressive neurodegenerative disease, and the diagnosis of the disease is possible at an early stage when the patient remains independent and the cognitive symptoms are still mild. The core clinical criteria for AD dementia will continue to be the cornerstone of the diagnosis in clinical practice, but new diagnostic proposals[4,10] advise inclusion of evidence from pathophysiologic

Table 2
Recommendations from the National Institute of Aging on diagnostic guidelines for AD by using biomarkers

	Diagnosis of AD at the MCI Stage		
	MCI Criteria Incorporating Biomarkers		
Diagnostic Category	Biomarker Probability of AD Cause	Aβ (PET or CSF)	Neuronal Injury (tau, FDG, sMR Imaging)
MCI: core clinical criteria	Uninformative	Conflicting/ indeterminate/ untested	Conflicting/ indeterminate/ untested
MCI caused by AD: intermediate likelihood	Intermediate	Positive Untested	Untested Positive
MCI caused by AD: high likelihood	Highest	Positive	Positive
MCI unlikely to be caused by AD	Lowest	Negative	Negative
	Diagnosis of AD at the Dementia Stage		
	AD Dementia Criteria Incorporating Biomarkers		
Diagnostic Category	Biomarker Probability of AD Cause	Aβ (PET or CSF)	Neuronal Injury (CSF tau, FDG-PET, sMR Imaging)
Probable AD dementia			
Based on clinical criteria	Uninformative	Unavailable, conflicting, or indeterminate	Unavailable, conflicting, or indeterminate
With 3 levels of evidence of AD pathophysiologic process	Intermediate	Unavailable or indeterminate	Positive
	Intermediate	Positive	Unavailable or indeterminate
	High	Positive	Positive
Possible AD dementia (atypical clinical presentation)			
Based on clinical criteria	Uninformative	Unavailable, conflicting, or indeterminate	Unavailable, conflicting, or indeterminate
With evidence of AD pathophysiologic process	High but does not rule out second cause	Positive	Positive
Dementia unlikely to be caused by AD	Lowest	Negative	Negative

Abbreviations: Aβ, amyloid β peptide; sMR imaging, structural MR imaging.
From Albert MS, Dekosky ST, Dickson D, et al. The diagnosis of mild cognitive impairment due to Alzheimer's disease: recommendations from the National Institute on Aging-Alzheimer's Association workgroups on diagnostic guidelines for Alzheimer's disease. Alzheimers Dement 2011;7:278; with permission [Diagnosis of AD at the MCI Stage]; and McKhann GM, Knopman DS, Chertkow H, et al. The diagnosis of dementia due to Alzheimer's disease: recommendations from the National Institute on Aging-Alzheimer's Association workgroups on diagnostic guidelines for Alzheimer's disease. Alzheimers Dement 2011;7:267; with permission [Diagnosis of AD at the Dementia Stage].

biomarker(s) to enhance the specificity of the diagnosis of AD dementia.

Concerning the interpretation of biomarkers in clinical practice, the recent recommendations from the NIA-AA[11] differ in some points from those of the IWG (Box 1, Tables 1 and 2).[4] The NIA-AA criteria propose the division of biomarkers into 2 major categories: (1) the biomarkers of Ab accumulation, that is, abnormal tracer retention on amyloid PET imaging and low CSF Ab; and (2) the biomarkers of neuronal degeneration or injury, that is, increased CSF tau (both total and phosphorylated tau), decreased FDG uptake on PET in a specific topographic pattern involving temporoparietal cortex, and atrophy on structural MR imaging, again in a specific topographic pattern, involving mainly medial temporal lobes and parietal cortices.[11] The NIA-AA criteria are described in 2 phases, according to the severity of the disease. In the symptomatic predementia (MCI) phase, biomarkers are used to establish the underlying cause of the clinical deficit. Different terminology is proposed for classifying individuals with MCI caused by AD with varying levels of certainty (see Table 1). In the dementia phase, biomarkers are used to assess the level of certainty of the underlying AD pathophysiologic process in a given patient.

In the proposals of the IWG criteria,[4,5] the diagnosis relies on (1) a major clinical criterion, which is based on the identification of a predominant episodic memory impairment, with evidence of a progressive amnestic syndrome of the hippocampal type; and (2) evidence of in vivo markers of AD, which can include CSF biomarkers (Ab, T-tau, P-tau), retention of specific PET amyloid tracers, medial temporal lobe atrophy on MR imaging, and/or temporal/parietal hypometabolism on FDG-PET. The diagnosis of AD can also be established in cases of proven AD autosomal dominant mutation. This working group[4] categorizes AD biomarkers as (1) pathophysiologic markers, including CSF biomarkers and PiB-PET, which correspond with the 2 causal degenerative processes that characterize Alzheimer's pathology (the amyloidosis path to neuritic plaques and the tauopathy path to neurofibrillary tangles); and (2) topographic markers that correspond with the downstream markers of neurodegeneration of the NIA-AA criteria, including MR imaging atrophy and FDG-PET, which assess the less specific downstream brain changes that correlate with the regional distribution of Alzheimer's pathology. Concerning the early (predementia) stage of AD, the new lexicon suggests using the term prodromal AD. To avoid confusion, the term MCI should be restricted to individuals who deviate from the clinicobiological phenotype of prodromal AD because they have memory symptoms that are not characteristic of AD or they are biomarker negative (or not available).[4]

Moreover, focal atypical presentation of AD, such as posterior cortical atrophy and logopenic aphasia, have been described in neuropathologic studies.[59] By using physiopathologic markers, such as CSF biomarkers and ^{11}C-PiB-PET, it is now possible to identify in vivo an underlying process similar to that observed in typical AD.[45,55,56] It is proposed that these clinical presentations, without predominant amnesia, should be called atypical AD.[4]

The clinical validity of these new diagnostic criteria is currently being discussed. Extensive work on biomarker standardization is needed before widespread adoption of these recommendations at any stage of the disease. No cutoff or normal/pathologic threshold is clearly defined for each biomarker. Much additional work needs to be done to validate the application of biomarkers as they are proposed in the published articles. Moreover, there is a need for a decisional algorithm for the clinical diagnosis that would guide clinicians in the choice of an invasive investigation such as CSF biomarkers or an expensive examination such as PET imaging.

REFERENCES

1. McKhann G, Drachman D, Folstein M, et al. Clinical diagnosis of Alzheimer's disease: report of the NINCDS-ADRDA Work Group under the auspices of Department of Health and Human Services Task Force on Alzheimer's Disease. Neurology 1984;34: 939–44.
2. Ballard C, Gauthier S, Corbett A, et al. Alzheimer's disease. Lancet 2011;377(9770):1019–31.
3. Blacker D, Albert MS, Bassett SS, et al. Reliability and validity of NINCDS-ADRDA criteria for Alzheimer's disease. The National Institute of Mental Health Genetics Initiative. Arch Neurol 1994;51: 1198–204.
4. Dubois B, Feldman HH, Jacova C, et al. Revising the definition of Alzheimer's disease: a new lexicon. Lancet Neurol 2010;9:1118–27.
5. Dubois B, Feldman HH, Jacova C, et al. Research criteria for the diagnosis of Alzheimer's disease: revising the NINCDS-ADRDA criteria. Lancet Neurol 2007;6:734–46.
6. Bouwman FH, Verwey NA, Klein M, et al. New research criteria for the diagnosis of Alzheimer's disease applied in a memory clinic population. Dement Geriatr Cogn Disord 2010;30:1–7.
7. de Jager CA, Honey TE, Birks J, et al. Retrospective evaluation of revised criteria for the diagnosis of

Alzheimer's disease using a cohort with post-mortem diagnosis. Int J Geriatr Psychiatry 2010;25(10):988–97.

8. Schoonenboom NS, van der Flier WM, Blankenstein MA, et al. CSF and MRI markers independently contribute to the diagnosis of Alzheimer's disease. Neurobiol Aging 2008;29:669–75.

9. Albert MS, Dekosky ST, Dickson D, et al. The diagnosis of mild cognitive impairment due to Alzheimer's disease: recommendations from the National Institute on Aging-Alzheimer's Association workgroups on diagnostic guidelines for Alzheimer's disease. Alzheimers Dement 2011;7:270–9.

10. DeKosky ST, Carrillo MC, Phelps C, et al. Revision of the criteria for Alzheimer's disease: a symposium. Alzheimers Dement 2011;7:e1–12.

11. Jack CR Jr, Albert MS, Knopman DS, et al. Introduction to the recommendations from the National Institute on Aging-Alzheimer's Association workgroups on diagnostic guidelines for Alzheimer's disease. Alzheimers Dement 2011;7:257–62.

12. McKhann GM, Knopman DS, Chertkow H, et al. The diagnosis of dementia due to Alzheimer's disease: recommendations from the National Institute on Aging-Alzheimer's Association workgroups on diagnostic guidelines for Alzheimer's disease. Alzheimers Dement 2011;7:263–9.

13. Sperling RA, Aisen PS, Beckett LA, et al. Toward defining the preclinical stages of Alzheimer's disease: recommendations from the National Institute on Aging-Alzheimer's Association workgroups on diagnostic guidelines for Alzheimer's disease. Alzheimers Dement 2011;7:280–92.

14. Braak H, Braak E. Neuropathological stageing of Alzheimer-related changes. Acta Neuropathol 1991; 82:239–59.

15. Dubois B, Albert ML. Amnestic MCI or prodromal Alzheimer's disease? Lancet Neurol 2004;3:246–8.

16. Buschke H, Sliwinski MJ, Kuslansky G, et al. Diagnosis of early dementia by the double memory test: encoding specificity improves diagnostic sensitivity and specificity. Neurology 1997;48:989–97.

17. Grober E, Buschke H, Crystal H, et al. Screening for dementia by memory testing. Neurology 1988;38:900–3.

18. Ivanoiu A, Adam S, Van der Linden M, et al. Memory evaluation with a new cued recall test in patients with mild cognitive impairment and Alzheimer's disease. J Neurol 2005;252:47–55.

19. Sarazin M, Berr C, De Rotrou J, et al. Amnestic syndrome of the medial temporal type identifies prodromal AD: a longitudinal study. Neurology 2007;69:1859–67.

20. Sarazin M, Chauvire V, Gerardin E, et al. The amnestic syndrome of hippocampal type in Alzheimer's disease: an MRI study. J Alzheimers Dis 2010;22:285–94.

21. Moscovitch M, Rosenbaum RS, Gilboa A, et al. Functional neuroanatomy of remote episodic, semantic and spatial memory: a unified account based on multiple trace theory. J Anat 2005;207:35–66.

22. Markesbery WR, Schmitt FA, Kryscio RJ, et al. Neuropathologic substrate of mild cognitive impairment. Arch Neurol 2006;63:38–46.

23. Pillon B, Blin J, Vidailhet M, et al. The neuropsychological pattern of corticobasal degeneration: comparison with progressive supranuclear palsy and Alzheimer's disease. Neurology 1995;45:1477–83.

24. Fossati P, Coyette F, Ergis AM, et al. Influence of age and executive functioning on verbal memory of inpatients with depression. J Affect Disord 2002; 68:261–71.

25. Traykov L, Baudic S, Raoux N, et al. Patterns of memory impairment and perseverative behavior discriminate early Alzheimer's disease from subcortical vascular dementia. J Neurol Sci 2005;229–230:75–9.

26. Lavenu I, Pasquier F, Lebert F, et al. Explicit memory in frontotemporal dementia: the role of medial temporal atrophy. Dement Geriatr Cogn Disord 1998;9:99–102.

27. Morris JC. The Clinical Dementia Rating (CDR): current version and scoring rules. Neurology 1993; 43:2412–4.

28. Blennow K, Hampel H, Weiner M, et al. Cerebrospinal fluid and plasma biomarkers in Alzheimer disease. Nat Rev Neurol 2010;6(3):131–44.

29. Frisoni GB, Fox NC, Jack CR Jr, et al. The clinical use of structural MRI in Alzheimer disease. Nat Rev Neurol 2010;6:67–77.

30. Lehericy S, Marjanska M, Mesrob L, et al. Magnetic resonance imaging of Alzheimer's disease. Eur Radiol 2007;17:347–62.

31. Yuan Y, Gu ZX, Wei WS. Fluorodeoxyglucose-positron-emission tomography, single-photon emission tomography, and structural MR imaging for prediction of rapid conversion to Alzheimer disease in patients with mild cognitive impairment: a meta-analysis. AJNR Am J Neuroradiol 2009;30:404–10.

32. McDonald CR, McEvoy LK, Gharapetian L, et al. Regional rates of neocortical atrophy from normal aging to early Alzheimer disease. Neurology 2009; 73:457–65.

33. Jack CR Jr, Dickson DW, Parisi JE, et al. Antemortem MRI findings correlate with hippocampal neuropathology in typical aging and dementia. Neurology 2002;58:750–7.

34. Korf ES, Wahlund LO, Visser PJ, et al. Medial temporal lobe atrophy on MRI predicts dementia in patients with mild cognitive impairment. Neurology 2004;63:94–100.

35. Scheltens P, Pasquier F, Weerts JG, et al. Qualitative assessment of cerebral atrophy on MRI: inter- and intra-observer reproducibility in dementia and normal aging. Eur Neurol 1997;37:95–9.

36. Chupin M, Gerardin E, Cuingnet R, et al. Fully automatic hippocampus segmentation and classification

in Alzheimer's disease and mild cognitive impairment applied on data from ADNI. Hippocampus 2009;19: 579–87.

37. Colliot O, Chetelat G, Chupin M, et al. Discrimination between Alzheimer disease, mild cognitive impairment, and normal aging by using automated segmentation of the hippocampus. Radiology 2008; 248:194–201.

38. Dougall NJ, Bruggink S, Ebmeier KP. Systematic review of the diagnostic accuracy of 99mTc-HMPAO-SPECT in dementia. Am J Geriatr Psychiatry 2004;12:554–70.

39. Habert MO, Horn JF, Sarazin M, et al. Brain perfusion SPECT with an automated quantitative tool can identify prodromal Alzheimer's disease among patients with mild cognitive impairment. Neurobiol Aging 2011;32:15–23.

40. Patwardhan MB, McCrory DC, Matchar DB, et al. Alzheimer disease: operating characteristics of PET–a meta-analysis. Radiology 2004;231:73–80.

41. Tapiola T, Alafuzoff I, Herukka SK, et al. Cerebrospinal fluid {beta}-amyloid 42 and tau proteins as biomarkers of Alzheimer-type pathologic changes in the brain. Arch Neurol 2009;66:382–9.

42. Hansson O, Zetterberg H, Buchhave P, et al. Association between CSF biomarkers and incipient Alzheimer's disease in patients with mild cognitive impairment: a follow-up study. Lancet Neurol 2006; 5:228–34.

43. Buerger K, Ewers M, Pirttila T, et al. CSF phosphorylated tau protein correlates with neocortical neurofibrillary pathology in Alzheimer's disease. Brain 2006;129:3035–41.

44. de Souza LC, Chupin M, Lamari F, et al. CSF tau markers are correlated with hippocampal volume in Alzheimer's disease. Neurobiol Aging 2011. DOI:10.1016/j.neurobiolaging.2011.02.022. [Epub ahead of print].

45. de Souza LC, Lamari F, Belliard S, et al. Cerebrospinal fluid biomarkers in the differential diagnosis of Alzheimer's disease from other cortical dementias. J Neurol Neurosurg Psychiatry 2010;82:240–6.

46. Bian H, Van Swieten JC, Leight S, et al. CSF biomarkers in frontotemporal lobar degeneration with known pathology. Neurology 2008;70:1827–35.

47. Ikonomovic MD, Klunk WE, Abrahamson EE, et al. Post-mortem correlates of in vivo PiB-PET amyloid imaging in a typical case of Alzheimer's disease. Brain 2008;131:1630–45.

48. Fodero-Tavoletti MT, Rowe CC, McLean CA, et al. Characterization of PiB binding to white matter in Alzheimer disease and other dementias. J Nucl Med 2009;50:198–204.

49. Klunk WE, Engler H, Nordberg A, et al. Imaging brain amyloid in Alzheimer's disease with Pittsburgh Compound-B. Ann Neurol 2004;55:306–19.

50. Rabinovici GD, Jagust WJ. Amyloid imaging in aging and dementia: testing the amyloid hypothesis in vivo. Behav Neurol 2009;21:117–28.

51. Johnson KA, Gregas M, Becker JA, et al. Imaging of amyloid burden and distribution in cerebral amyloid angiopathy. Ann Neurol 2007;62:229–34.

52. Koivunen J, Scheinin N, Virta JR, et al. Amyloid PET imaging in patients with mild cognitive impairment: a 2-year follow-up study. Neurology 2011;76: 1085–90.

53. Okello A, Koivunen J, Edison P, et al. Conversion of amyloid positive and negative MCI to AD over 3 years: an 11C-PIB PET study. Neurology 2009;73:754–60.

54. Rabinovici GD, Jagust WJ, Furst AJ, et al. Abeta amyloid and glucose metabolism in three variants of primary progressive aphasia. Ann Neurol 2008; 64:388–401.

55. de Souza LC, Corlier F, Habert MO, et al. Similar amyloid-{beta} burden in posterior cortical atrophy and Alzheimer's disease. Brain 2011;134:2036–43.

56. Rosenbloom MH, Alkalay A, Agarwal N, et al. Distinct clinical and metabolic deficits in PCA and AD are not related to amyloid distribution. Neurology 2011;76:1789–96.

57. Edison P, Rowe CC, Rinne JO, et al. Amyloid load in Parkinson's disease dementia and Lewy body dementia measured with [11C]PIB positron emission tomography. J Neurol Neurosurg Psychiatry 2008; 79:1331–8.

58. Engler H, Santillo AF, Wang SX, et al. In vivo amyloid imaging with PET in frontotemporal dementia. Eur J Nucl Med Mol Imaging 2008;35:100–6.

59. Alladi S, Xuereb J, Bak T, et al. Focal cortical presentations of Alzheimer's disease. Brain 2007;130:2636–45.

Structural Neuroimaging in Aging and Alzheimer's Disease

Meike W. Vernooij, MD, PhD[a,b,*], Marion Smits, MD, PhD[a]

KEYWORDS

- Dementia • Alzheimer's disease
- Magnetic resonance (MR) imaging • Normal aging
- Brain • Atrophy • Neuroimaging

Structural neuroimaging in dementia has traditionally served the sole purpose of ruling out (treatable) disease as an alternative explanation for cognitive deterioration, for example a brain tumor or subdural hematoma. However, with more widespread use of magnetic resonance (MR) imaging and the development of more advanced imaging techniques (including diffusion-weighted and susceptibility-weighted imaging, positron emission tomography, or single-photon emission computed tomography), the role of neuroimaging in dementia has shifted gradually from exclusion of disease toward that of a highly valuable aid to the clinical diagnosis and subtyping of dementia.[1] To this end, MR imaging is preferred over computed tomography (CT), because it has the advantage of not only assessing (regional) atrophy (for which CT is sufficient) but also depicting other brain changes such as white matter lesions (WMLs) and microbleeds. Furthermore, there is increasing evidence showing that the pathologic process associated with dementia may begin decades before diagnosis. Detecting such preclinical changes by means of imaging could imply a major role for neuroimaging in risk stratification and early disease prevention. Yet, many brain changes seen in dementia also occur in middle-aged and elderly individuals who are

cognitively intact, and are considered part of the normal aging process. Distinguishing normal from abnormal aging is therefore a prerequisite when interpreting an imaging examination of an individual suspected of Alzheimer's disease (AD) or non-Alzheimer's dementia, and even more so when the goal of imaging shifts toward prediction of development of dementia. Structural MR imaging is the primary neuroimaging technique of choice in clinical practice to support the clinical diagnosis of dementia. This article focuses on structural MR neuroimaging in normal aging and in dementia, more specifically in AD. In the first part, normal versus pathologic brain aging is discussed, focusing on qualitative and quantitative MR imaging markers. In the second part, the role of MR imaging in the (differential) diagnosis of AD is reviewed.

PART I: STRUCTURAL IMAGING IN AGING

To recognize the abnormal, one needs to first know what is normal. With increasing age, the brain may show structural changes to varying degrees. Many of these brain changes overlap with the spectrum of disease present in dementia and AD, and there is a fine line between normal and pathologic brain

Funding support: None.
The authors have nothing to disclose.
[a] Department of Radiology, Erasmus MC University Medical Center, PO Box 2040, 3000 CA Rotterdam, The Netherlands
[b] Department of Epidemiology, Erasmus MC University Medical Center, PO Box 2040, 3000 CA Rotterdam, The Netherlands
* Corresponding author. Department of Radiology, Erasmus MC, PO Box 2040, 3000 CA Rotterdam, The Netherlands.
E-mail address: m.vernooij@erasmusmc.nl

neuroimaging.theclinics.com

aging. Moreover, even among those persons considered to age normally, there is a wide range, varying from successful brain aging (ie, retaining normal brain structure and volume up to high age) to the more typical aging or even near-pathologic brain aging (**Fig. 1**). Also, even although changes such as atrophy or WMLs are to a certain extent considered to be part of the normal aging spectrum, these have consistently been related to vascular risk factors. Furthermore, their presence may be accompanied by subtle cognitive deficits or even an increased risk of neurodegenerative or cerebrovascular disease. Studying the distribution and the time course of alterations that occur in the normal brain with aging is therefore important for understanding the mechanisms leading to these changes and for better characterization of neurologic disorders of which the risk increases with advancing age, such as dementia. Furthermore, because more clinical trials on therapy for AD are investigating imaging measures as surrogate markers for disease outcome, it becomes of particular importance to take into account the normal age-related brain changes that can be expected.

This section describes what changes are commonly found in the aging brain, to what extent these can be regarded as normal, and how these could be interpreted in the context of (suspected) AD.

A summary of common imaging findings in normal aging is presented in **Box 1**.

Brain Atrophy and Hippocampal Atrophy

Insight into changes of total brain volume with aging can be derived from various cross-sectional and longitudinal studies. Several automated image-processing tools have been developed to quantify total brain volume (**Box 2**), all with high levels of reproducibility.[7] Cross-sectional studies have consistently shown in non-demented persons older than 55 years that brain volumes are smaller with increasing age,[8,9] in persons with cardiovascular risk factors, and even more so when imaging findings consistent with cerebral small vessel disease are present.[9,10] When gray and white matter are studied separately, the rate of decline with age varies according to the age range studied. Several studies report a steady decline in gray matter from early adulthood onwards,[11–13] but others find that in elderly individuals, gray matter loss seems to become less prominent and that it is primarily white matter atrophy that causes the brain to shrink (**Fig. 4**).[9,14] There are few longitudinal studies that have examined changes in brain volume within individuals over time. For the purpose of comparison and to correct for head size differences, brain tissue volumes are generally expressed as percentage of intracranial volume. A mean rate of brain volume loss of 0.4% to 0.5% per year in normal middle-aged and elderly individuals has been described,[10,14] and double that rate (1.0%) in individuals who developed dementia during follow-up.[12] Yet, even among individuals remaining free of dementia, there is extensive evidence that total brain volume and separate gray/white matter volumes relate to cognitive performance in various cognitive domains.[9,15]

In the context of AD, hippocampal volume loss in normal aging is of particular interest. Manual

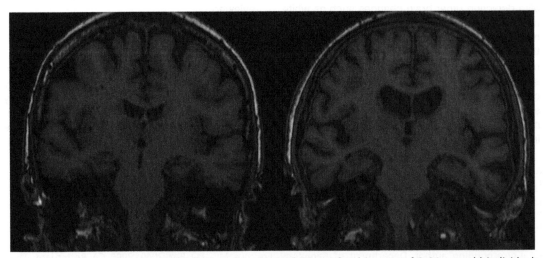

Fig. 1. Successful versus less-successful brain aging. Coronal T1-weighted images of 2 84-year-old individuals, both with normal Mini Mental State Examination scores. Yet, the brain of the individual on the left shows less atrophy compared with that of the individual on the right (total brain volume expressed as percentage of intracranial volume: 84% for the individual on the left vs 76% on the right).

Box 1
Summary of common brain MR imaging findings in aging

Brain atrophy

- Total brain volume: 0.4–0.5% brain tissue loss per year is normal, >1.0% is likely abnormal
- Hippocampus: volume loss 1.6%/y in normal individuals
- Normal volume loss in aging should be taken into account in clinical setting or in trials; reference data derived from normal population may be helpful

WMLs

- Punctiform or early confluent lesions (Fazekas score 0–2) in periventricular or subcortical distribution is generally normal in aging
- Confluent lesions are always abnormal (Fazekas score 3)
- MR imaging sequences such as diffusion tensor imaging (DTI) are more sensitive in detecting micro-structural changes in normal-appearing white matter

Cerebral microbleeds

- T2*-weighted MR imaging sequence needed for depiction
- Common in elderly individuals: prevalence more than 20% in persons older than 60 years
- (Strictly) lobar distribution linked to cerebral amyloid angiopathy (CAA) and AD
- Deep or infratentorial distribution related to hypertensive arteriolosclerosis
- New microbleeds develop yearly in 3%–7% of aging individuals

Silent brain infarcts

- Small lacunar strokes that are presumably without symptoms, but have been linked to subtle cognitive deficits and increased risk of stroke and dementia
- Present in 11%–28% of individuals older than 55 years

Enlarged perivascular spaces (EPVSs)

- Common around anterior commissure, in centrum semiovale, near vertex of the brain, and in hippocampus
- May be considered normal in most individuals but have also been linked to small vessel disease, cognitive deficits, and risk of dementia

---

outlining of hippocampal borders has long been the method of choice to obtain volumetric measures (for a detailed description, see Ref.[16]). Manual tracing is tedious, resource intensive, and prone to human error. These limitations become particularly relevant when large MR imaging data sets from population-based studies are to be analyzed, arguing for a need for automated measurements. Current automated methods, mainly atlas-based registration, have been shown to yield reliable and valid data,[17] and results are still improving.[18] Using automated segmentation, a longitudinal population-based study in 518 nondemented aging individuals showed a decline of 1.6% in hippocampal volume per year,[19] which is similar to a rate of 1.4% per year that was established/found among 200 healthy control individuals in a meta-analysis of AD case-control studies.[20] For comparison, the AD individuals in this meta-analysis had a mean decline in hippocampal volume of 4.7% per year. In the longitudinal study mentioned earlier, individuals who showed a larger rate of decline in hippocampal volume during follow-up more often developed dementia (the odds ratio to develop dementia was 2.3 per standard deviation of volume loss). Among those subjects who stayed free of dementia during follow-up, a faster decline in hippocampal volume was still related to worse performance on memory tests.[19]

These findings show that there seems to be a spectrum from normal aging to pathologic brain aging, rather than a distinct separation between healthy and diseased states. Furthermore, it implies that knowledge of normal rates of atrophy in aging is of importance for clinical trials in AD, when the rate of brain atrophy or hippocampal atrophy is used as a surrogate marker of disease progression, but also in a clinical setting taking into account a patient's age is important to

---

Box 2
Automated methods to measure brain atrophy

Brain atrophy has originally been assessed using visual rating scales (eg, global cortical atrophy [GCA] scale, see **Table 1**), yielding crude and observer-dependent measures, which are less useful for assessment of change over time. More recently developed automated algorithms allow for absolute quantification of many features, increasing the usefulness of volumetric measurements to distinguish normal from abnormal aging. These automated methods can be grossly divided into segmentation-based analyses and registration-based analyses. For a more detailed discussion of these methods, see Ref.[2]

Segmentation-based analysis

For tissue segmentation, T1-weighted images, preferably with isotropic voxel size, are most often used as input. Freely available segmentation algorithms that are frequently used are those incorporated in the SPM (http://www.fil.ion.ucl.ac.uk/spm/) and FSL software packages (http://www.fmrib.ox.ac.uk/fsl/). These segmentation processes yield for each voxel the probability of belonging to a certain tissue class (gray matter, white matter, cerebral spinal fluid [CSF] or background). A typical segmentation result is shown in **Fig. 2**. These probability maps can then be used to estimate tissue volumes on an individual level or to perform group-wise analyses on a voxel level (voxel-based morphometry[3]). A disadvantage of most tissue segmentation algorithms is that these are not able to segment WMLs. To this end, a fully automated algorithm developed on fluid-attenuated inversion recovery (FLAIR) images has been described recently.[4]

Registration-based analysis

In the process of image registration, 1 image is brought in anatomic correspondence with another image, by a method of registration that uses a variable amount of degrees of freedom (as a rule of thumb, using more degrees of freedom is more time-intensive but yields a better registration). Applying registration methods to scans from a single individual collected at 2 different time points enables assessment of change in brain volume over time as depicted in **Fig. 3**. Methods like SIENA within the FSL package (http://www.fmrib.ox.ac.uk/fsl/siena/index.html)[5] or the brain boundary shift integral method[6] both directly visualize change in brain volume over time.

---

determine whether they show an abnormal degree of brain tissue loss. For this use, reference data on brain tissue volumes derived from a normal aging population are of great value (**Fig. 5**).

WMLs and White Matter Microstructure

In elderly individuals, focal white matter abnormalities occur frequently, seen on CT as mildly hypodense areas and on T2-weighted MR imaging or FLAIR images as hyperintense foci in the white matter (**Fig. 6**). Commonly used terminology includes WMLs, white matter hyperintensities, or age-related white matter changes. WML load increases with age (**Fig. 7**) and typically shows a periventricular or subcortical distribution (**Box 3**, **Fig. 10**). Although the pathogenesis remains unclear, histopathologic studies point toward hypoxic/ischemic injury caused by hypoperfusion as the underlying cause.[26] This theory is further supported by findings that classic cardiovascular risk factors, such as hypertension, smoking, and diabetes, are all related to the presence and progression of WMLs.[26,27] Although longitudinal

Table 1
Visual rating scale of GCA

	Degree of Atrophy	Gyri	Sulci
GCA = 0	None	Normal volume	Normal width
GCA = 1	Mild (may be considered normal in the elderly)	Normal	Some opening of sulci
GCA = 2	Moderate	Reduced	Enlarged
GCA = 3	Severe	Severely reduced (knife blade)	Severely enlarged

Data from Pasquier F, Leys D, Weerts JG, et al. Inter- and intraobserver reproducibility of cerebral atrophy assessment on MR imaging scans with hemispheric infarcts. Eur Neurol 1996;36(5):268–72.

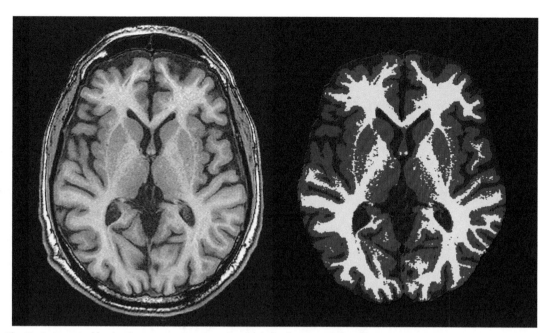

Fig. 2. Automated brain tissue segmentation. On the left, the T1-weighted image used as input and on the right, the segmentation result in which each voxel has been labeled according to its tissue class.

studies have shown that lesion load in presumed healthy persons is related to an increased risk of stroke, dementia, and death,[27,28] cross-sectional reports show only a weak correlation between WML and symptoms, such as cognitive deficits.[27] This finding may be related to the fact that the

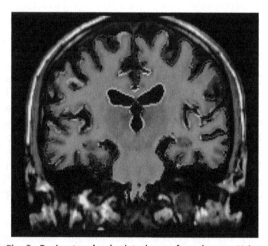

Fig. 3. Brain atrophy depicted as surface change. Using SIENA,[5] 2 brain scans from a single individual obtained at different time points (interval 3 years) are segmented into brain and nonbrain tissue and then registered to each other. The resulting image shows regional decrease in volume (*in blue*) or increase (*in red*) over time. (Image kindly prepared by Dr Renske de Boer.)

underlying extent of tissue disease (ie, myelin loss or axonal damage) may differ between several kinds of lesions that all have a similar appearance on MR imaging. Furthermore, WMLs likely mark underlying vasculopathy that causes changes in normal-appearing brain tissue that are not visible on conventional MR imaging. Various advanced MR techniques have emerged in recent years to assess these hidden abnormalities in apparently normal brain tissue. Examples are magnetic transfer ratio, spectroscopy, or T1 and T2 relaxation measures, the use of which has been described extensively in relation to white matter diseases such as multiple sclerosis.[29] A more recent emerging technique is DTI, which enables the quantification of random movement of water molecules in brain tissue, by applying strong magnetic gradients in various directions.[30] Normal brain tissue, especially white matter, hinders the degree and direction of random diffusion because of its highly structured fiber organization. With loss of microstructural integrity of white matter, diffusion properties change to a measurable extent. Parameters derived from DTI that are used commonly to quantify tissue integrity are mean diffusivity (MD, magnitude of diffusion) and fractional anisotropy (FA, degree of anisotropy of diffusion). With increasing age, MD has been consistently found to increase in normal-appearing white matter, and FA to decrease.[31,32] These changes were found to relate more to WML load and atrophy than to

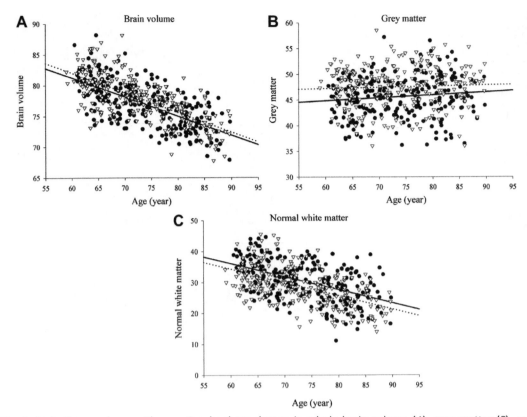

Fig. 4. Brain tissue volume with age. Graphs show change in whole brain volume (*A*), gray matter (*B*), and normal white matter (*C*), as function of age, expressed as percentage of intracranial volume. (*Reprinted from* Ikram MA, Vrooman HA, Vernooij MW, et al. Brain tissue volumes in the general elderly population. The Rotterdam Scan Study. Neurobiol Aging 2008;29(6):886.)

age in itself (**Fig. 11**),[33] thus supporting the idea that WMLs merely represent the tip of the iceberg and that damage to the white matter is more widespread than can be appreciated on conventional MR images. More importantly, DTI changes in normal-appearing brain tissue relate to cognitive function in community-dwelling elderly individuals, independent of degree of brain atrophy or WML load,[34,35] suggesting that DTI more sensitively detects clinically significant white matter changes and that this measure may complement traditional volumetric measures. More recent approaches have been directed toward quantification of DTI parameters in distinct white matter tracts that can be identified using tractography methods (**Fig. 12**). These advances will yield tract-specific information on diffusion properties, which is of relevance to the hypothesis that cognitive decline may in part be caused by disconnection of specific cortical-subcortical connections.[36] It is expected that such methods may aid in detecting more subtle changes in white matter disease over time, which could for example be used as a surrogate marker to evaluate new therapies in clinical trials. Again,

reference estimates derived from aging individuals are essential to interpret findings in a clinical setting.

Cerebral Microbleeds

Cerebral microbleeds are small brain hemorrhages that are presumed to result from leakage of blood cells from damaged small vessel walls. They were first detected on MR imaging only in the mid-1990s, as MR imaging sequences sensitive to blood-breakdown products became available (eg, T2*-weighted gradient-echo technique), which are essential for microbleed detection (**Fig. 13**).[37] Histologically, these small black dots on MR imaging represent hemosiderin-laden macrophages that are clustered around small vessels (**Fig. 14**). The choice of field strength, sequence parameters (particularly echo time), and postprocessing (eg, susceptibility-weighted imaging technique) have all been found to have a major influence on the detection rate of cerebral microbleeds.[38–40] With these advances in imaging, the prevalence of microbleeds has been estimated to be more than 20% in persons aged 60 years and

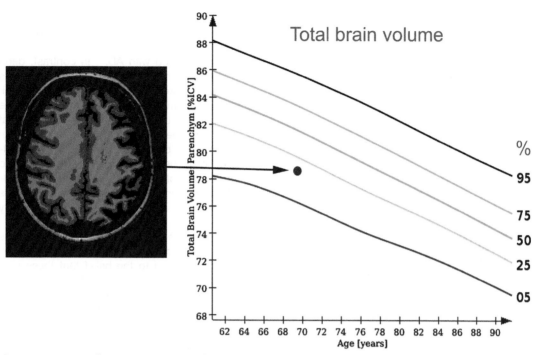

Fig. 5. Normative reference data as an aid for clinical diagnosis. A brain tissue segmentation result is shown (*left*). The brain volume derived from this segmentation can be compared with reference curves derived from the general aging population (*graph*). The graph depicts the percentile lines (5%–95%) for brain volume as percentage of intracranial volume, as a function of age (x-axis). The measurement of the individual on the left is plotted in the graph as a gray circle. (*Courtesy of* Dr Bas Jasperse and Dr Marcel Koek.)

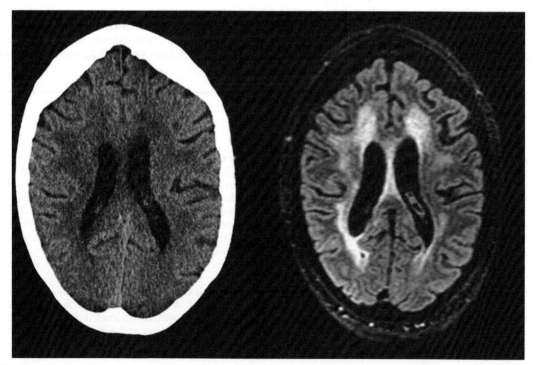

Fig. 6. WMLs seen as hypodense regions on CT (*left*) and as hyperintensities on FLAIR MR imaging (*right*).

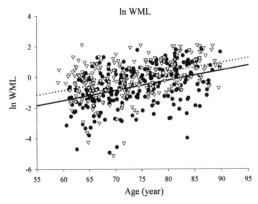

Fig. 7. Graph showing increase in WML volume as function of age. Note that WML volume was ln-transformed because of skewness of untransformed measure. (*Reprinted from* Ikram MA, Vrooman HA, Vernooij MW, et al. Brain tissue volumes in the general elderly population. The Rotterdam Scan Study. Neurobiol Aging 2008;29(6):886; with permission.)

older, increasing to nearly 40% in those older than 80 years.[41] Microbleed location is generally divided into deep (ie, basal ganglia, thalamus) and infratentorial versus lobar brain regions (Fig. 15). In the aging population, microbleeds in lobar locations share apolipoprotein E (APOE) ε4 genotype as a common risk factor with CAA and AD, suggestive of a potential link between vascular and amyloid neuropathology.[41,42] This link has further been corroborated by the finding that topography of lobar microbleeds in community-dwelling elderly individuals follows the same posterior distribution as is known from amyloid disease in CAA and AD.[43] Furthermore, recent reports show that

presence of microbleeds, and particularly those in lobar locations, relates to worse cognitive function, both in healthy elderly individuals[44,45] and in patients diagnosed with AD.[46] In contrast, deep or infratentorial microbleeds in aging individuals are primarily linked to classic cardiovascular risk factors and are more likely caused by hypertensive vasculopathy.[41] Longitudinal studies indicate that incident microbleeds commonly occur over time: annually, 3% of presumed healthy elderly individuals develop new microbleeds, increasing to more than 7% of those who already have microbleeds at baseline.[47] In comparison, these rates are doubled in patients attending a memory clinic.[48]

The increasing evidence that microbleeds reflect both vascular disease as well as amyloid angiopathy has led to the belief that these may well represent the missing link between the vascular and amyloid hypotheses in the pathogenesis of AD, which is further elaborated on in part II of this article.

Silent Brain Infarcts

Small lacunar infarcts (Fig. 16) are often found on brain MR imaging in the aging population without previous history of stroke and these have therefore been named silent brain infarcts. Population-based studies have estimated the prevalence of silent infarcts on MR imaging to range from 11% to 28% for those aged 55 years and older.[49] These estimates are likely to vary as a result of large heterogeneity in MR imaging parameters and diagnostic criteria, and the difficulty in distinguishing lacunar infarcts from EPVSs.[50] As expected, silent

---

Box 3
Assessment of WML load

Visual rating

A large variety of visual rating scales is available to assess the amount and distribution of WMLs. Easiest to use (and therefore most commonly applied in clinical care) is the Fazekas rating scale,[21] which describes WML load separately for periventricular and deep WMLs in a 4-step scale (score 0–3; Fig. 8). A general interpretation of the Fazekas scores is that score 1 (punctiform lesions only) is normal for most individuals, even those aged less than 65 years. Score 2 is considered abnormal for persons aged 70 years and less, whereas score 3 (confluent lesions) should always be viewed as abnormal. The Age-Related White Matter Changes (ARWMC) scale[22] also applies a 4-step scale but on a larger number of regions (Table 2). A more elaborate and semiquantitative scale is that of Scheltens and colleagues.[23]

Automated segmentation

Despite the ease of visual rating, studies have shown that there is considerable interrater reliability for the use of these scales, especially concerning WML progression.[24,25] Alternatively, WML volume can be quantified by manually outlining all lesions and summing these to obtain volumetric measures that may better capture change over time. Yet, this practice is time-consuming and may still be prone to human error. An observer-free and reproducible assessment of WML load may better be obtained by fully automated tissue segmentation procedures (for an example, see Ref.[4]) (Fig. 9).

Table 2		
ARWMC rating scale for WMLs on MR imaging and CT		
WMLs		
0		No lesions (may include symmetric, well-defined caps or bands)
1		Focal lesions
2		Beginning confluence of lesions
3		Diffuse involvement of the entire region, with or without involvement of U-fibers
Basal ganglia lesions		
0		No lesions
1		1 focal lesion ($\geq$5 mm)
2		>1 focal lesion
3		Confluent lesions

White matter changes on MR imaging are defined as ill-defined hyperintensities $\geq$5 mm on both T2 and proton density/FLAIR images, and on CT as ill-defined and moderately hypodense areas of $\geq$5 mm. Lesions are scored for left and right hemisphere separately in the following brain areas: frontal, parieto-occipital, temporal, infratentorial/cerebellum, and basal ganglia (striatum, globus pallidus, thalamus, internal/external capsule, and insula). For each of these regions, the sum score of left and right hemisphere therefore is from 0 to 6.

Data from Wahlund LO, Barkhof F, Fazekas F, et al. A new rating scale for age-related white matter changes applicable to MRI and CT. Stroke 2001;32(6):1318–22.

brain infarct prevalence is higher with increase in age and with risk factors also known to be related to clinical stroke, such as hypertension, atrial fibrillation, carotid intima-media thickness, and increased plasma homocysteine.[49] More recent publications also point toward kidney disease as an important risk factor,[51] which indicates that cerebral small vessel disease may be a reflection of more systemic vascular damage. Furthermore, silent brain infarcts show a strong association with WML load, again supporting small vessel disease as a common underlying pathophysiology. This finding has been further substantiated by a link between retinal microvascular abnormalities and both lacunar infarcts and WMLs in a large sample of aging individuals.[52] Despite their name, the fact that silent infarct presence has been related to subtle cognitive deficits and more than doubles risk of stroke and dementia (in particular AD[49]) suggests that these are neither silent nor innocuous.

EPVSs

Perivascular spaces, also named Virchow-Robin spaces, are extensions of the subarachnoid space that accompany vessels entering the brain parenchyma. EPVSs commonly occur around arteries in the substantia perforata, in the region of the anterior commissure, in the centrum semiovale, or near the vertex of the brain (**Fig. 17**). Their typical imaging appearance is that of sharply demarcated dotlike or linear CSF-filled spaces. Prominent or dilated perivascular spaces can be seen at all ages, even in the very young,[53] in whom they are considered a normal finding. However, with aging, EPVSs may become more prominent[54] and have been associated with presence of silent brain infarcts and WML load.[54,55] This association with cerebral small vessel disease was further supported by recent evidence that in a large population-based sample of elderly individuals, those with hypertension had more prominent perivascular spaces compared with normotensives.[54]

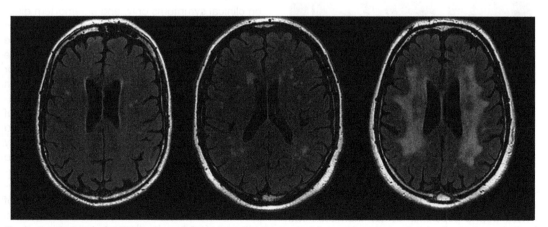

Fig. 8. Fazekas scale for WMLs. From left to right, Fazekas scale 1 (punctiform lesions), 2 (early confluent lesions), and 3 (confluent lesions) (not shown: score 0 = no lesions).

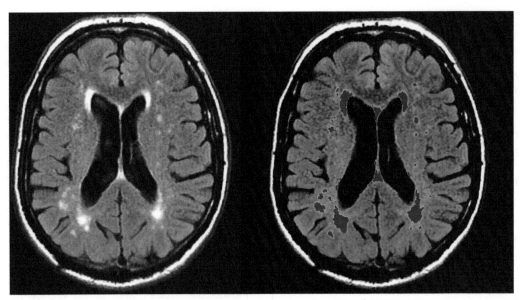

Fig. 9. WML segmentation result. Using automated segmentation algorithms,[4] WMLs can be segmented on FLAIR images (*left*), yielding labeled voxels (*right*) that can be summed to quantify WML load or be used to analyze regional distribution of WMLs. (*Courtesy of* Dr Renske de Boer.)

More importantly, there are suggestions that EPVSs relate to subtle cognitive deficits[56] and even increased risk of dementia, independent of WML volume and presence of brain infarcts.[57] One peculiar location of EPVSs is the hippocampal

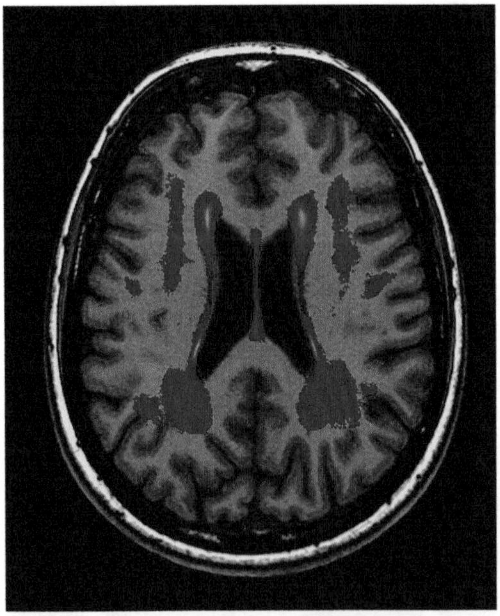

Fig. 10. Common locations of WMLs. Image represents a probability map (thresholded at 0.02–0.9), derived from a population of 567 individuals with mean age of 67 years (range 60–88 years). (Image kindly prepared by Dr Renske de Boer.)

area,[58] where they may be named hippocampal cavities or hippocampal cysts (see **Fig. 17**); some consider these to represent failure of closure of the hippocampal sulcus rather than EPVSs.[59] Irrespective of their presumed origin and notwithstanding the interesting location, no clear role has been attributed to the presence of these cyst-like lesions in the hippocampal region.

PART II: STRUCTURAL NEUROIMAGING IN AD

Until recently, the diagnostic criteria for AD, most notably those set out by the National Institute of Neurologic Communicative Disorders and Stroke–Alzheimer's Disease and Related Disorders Association (NINCDS-ADRDA),[60] were based on clinical symptoms only, and antemortem diagnostic certainty was limited to probable AD. In the 2011 revision, the NINCDS-ADRDA criteria include structural and functional biomarkers to provide evidence of AD pathophysiologic process[61] for research purposes. Early diagnosis of AD even with the revised NINCDS-ADRDA criteria is by definition impossible, because the presence of a dementia syndrome is required. Dubois and colleagues[1] propose to discard this severity threshold and reserve the term AD for the in vivo clinicobiological expression of the disease, encompassing the whole severity spectrum of its clinical course. Within this framework, the diagnosis of AD requires the presence of the core diagnostic criterion of early episodic memory impairment, as well as a minimum of 1 supporting biomarker,

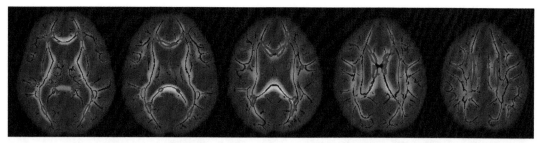

Fig. 11. Decrease in FA in normal-appearing white matter in aging individuals. Images represent skeletonized white matter (for details, see http://fsl.fmrib.ox.ac.uk/fsl/tbss/). In red are regions that show significant decrease in FA with increasing age. (*Adapted from* Vernooij MW, de Groot M, van der Lugt A, et al. White matter atrophy and lesion formation explain the loss of structural integrity of white matter in aging. Neuroimage 2008; 43(3):472.)

derived from structural MR imaging, CSF, metabolic imaging, or genetics.[1] The distinction between possible and probable AD, as made with the NINCDS-ADRDA criteria, is no longer made; instead a distinction is made between typical and atypical AD. Although these criteria are not yet widely accepted as clinical diagnostic criteria, they emphasize the increasing diagnostic role for structural neuroimaging in AD.

Typical Presentation of AD

The radiological hallmark finding of AD is cortical atrophy caused by neuronal degeneration and loss. Atrophy is diffuse, but more prominent in the temporal and parietal lobes, with the hippocampus most severely and disproportionately affected

(Fig. 18). The primary motor and sensory cortices are relatively spared until late in the disease. Findings are bilateral and generally symmetric, but a certain degree of asymmetry may occur. White matter volume is also reduced, presumed to be secondary to Wallerian degeneration after cortical neuronal cell death. Ventricles and sulci are consequently also enlarged. Widening of the CSF spaces is most prominent surrounding the entorhinal cortex and the hippocampus (ie, the temporal horn and the choroid fissure). The temporospatial distribution of atrophy follows that of the histopathologic characteristics of AD. Neurofibrillary tangles and neuropil threads first appear in the transentorhinal and entorhinal areas (parahippocampal gyrus), increasing in density during the course of the disease and appearing in the hippocampus,

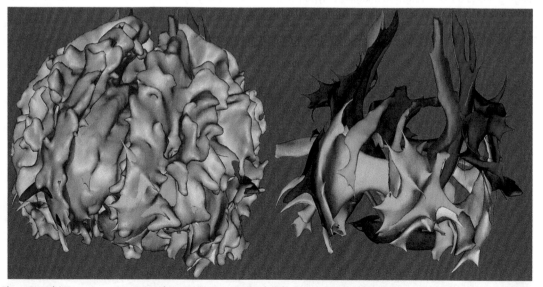

Fig. 12. White matter tractography. Postprocessing of diffusion tensor images using tractography algorithms enables isolation of separate white matter tracts, depicted in color (example shown for individual on *left*, brain surface rendering, on right, isolated tracts). (Image kindly prepared by Dr Marius de Groot.)

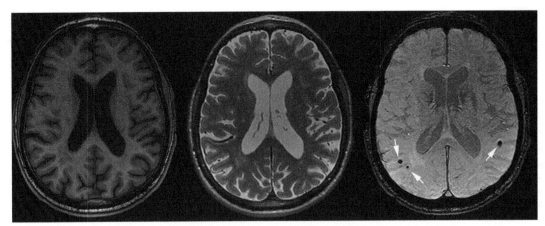

Fig. 13. Microbleed imaging. T1-weighted (*left*), T2-weighted (*middle*), and T2*-weighted (*right*) images. Cerebral microbleeds, depicted by arrows, are visualized only on the T2*-weighted image and not on the T1-weighted or T2-weighted images. The T2*-weighted image is susceptible to paramagnetic properties of hemosiderin, causing the microbleeds to appear as black dots of signal loss.

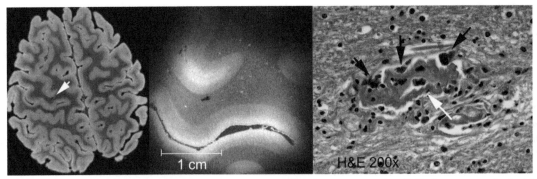

Fig. 14. Radiologic-pathologic correlation of cerebral microbleeds on MR imaging (3 T). Postmortem brain MR imaging shows on T2*-weighted imaging a hypointense focus on the gray-white matter interface (*white arrow*). MR image in the middle of the isolated tissue block containing this hypointense focus. Pathologic analysis of this tissue block (hematoxylin and eosin stain) shows macrophages containing hemosiderin (*black arrows*), confirming that the hypointense lesion on MR imaging is compatible with a microbleed.

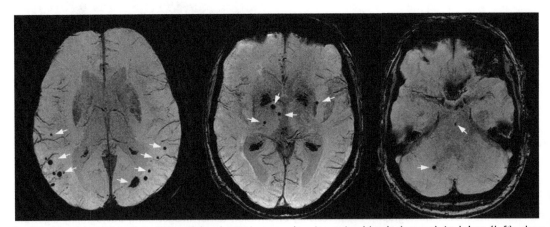

Fig. 15. Microbleed location. T2*-weighted MR images showing microbleeds (*arrows*) in lobar (*left*), deep (*middle*), and infratentorial (*right*) locations.

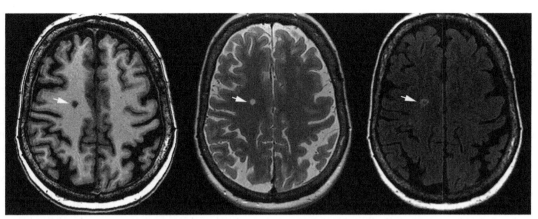

Fig. 16. Silent brain infarct. T1-weighted (*left*), T2-weighted (*right*), and FLAIR images showing a lacunar infarct (*arrow*) in the left centrum semiovale in an asymptomatic 72-year-old man. Note that the lacune has signal intensity similar to CSF on all sequences and furthermore shows a hyperintense rim on the FLAIR sequence, indicating gliosis.

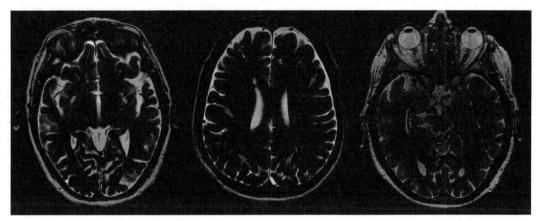

Fig. 17. T2-weighted images of prominent perivascular spaces (*red arrows*) in the region of the anterior commissure (*left*), in the centrum semiovale (*middle*) and the hippocampus (*right*).

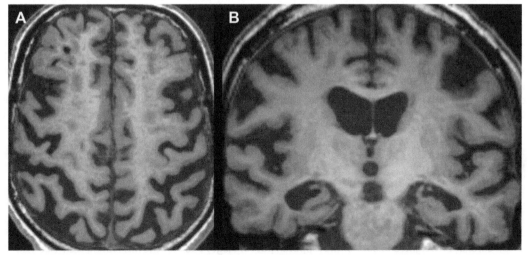

Fig. 18. Seventy-six-year-old man with AD. Transverse (*A*) and coronal (*B*) T1-weighted images show cortical atrophy, more prominently in the parietal than in the frontal lobe (*A*), with disproportionate hippocampal atrophy (*B*).

further progressing from the limbic system to the temporal and parietal association cortices and eventually to the entire neocortex.[62] Accordingly, focal entorhinal cortical and hippocampal atrophy occurs early and remains the most prominent feature in the disease process.[63]

Hippocampal atrophy

Multiple studies confirm hippocampal volume loss in patients with AD compared with healthy controls.[64,65] Sensitivity and specificity in distinguishing patients with AD from healthy controls are in the range of 85% and 88%, respectively.[65] Findings regarding entorhinal cortex atrophy are similar, but not more accurate than hippocampal atrophy to distinguish patients with AD from healthy controls.[66]

Although atrophy of the medial temporal lobe is commonly seen in patients with AD (70%–95%), it is also frequently seen in patients with minor cognitive impairment (MCI), although the frequency is lower (60%–80%) and extent of hippocampal atrophy is less pronounced.[67] However, sensitivity and specificity of hippocampal atrophy to identify prodromal AD are only in the range of 70%, indicating limited clinical usefulness.[1] Adding entorhinal cortex measurements may improve accuracy,[65] although findings are inconsistent.[1] More recently, studies have focused on using hippocampal shape, rather than volume, to predict AD. Preliminary results are promising in that they show that hippocampal shape provides additional predictive value over hippocampal volume.[68,69]

Hippocampal atrophy may be seen in other conditions, such as hippocampal sclerosis, mesial temporal sclerosis and temporal lobe epilepsy, ischemic insults to the hippocampus, and herpes simplex encephalitis.[1] Furthermore, hippocampal atrophy is common in other types of dementia, such as dementia with Lewy bodies (DLB), frontotemporal dementia (FTD), and the Heidenhain variant of Creutzfeldt-Jakob disease (CJD).[63] Consequently, diagnostic accuracy to distinguish AD from other dementias is considerably lower than from healthy controls.

Medial temporal atrophy rating scale

The most commonly used and well-validated method to assess hippocampal atrophy is the medial temporal atrophy (MTA) scale.[70] This 5-point visual rating scale ranging from normal (score = 0) to severe atrophy (score = 4) assesses 3 easily recognizable structures on coronal MR images: the width of the choroidal fissure, the width of the temporal horn, and the height of the hippocampal body (**Fig. 19, Table 3**). A score of 0 to 1 may be considered normal in persons younger than 75 years, whereas a score of 2 may still be considered normal at older than 75 years. The MTA scale correlates well with both linear[71] and volumetric[71,72] measurements of the hippocampus and has reasonable interobserver agreement, with best results obtained when the scale is dichotomized (MTA = 0–1 vs MTA = 2–4).[73] In the absence of automated algorithms it is less time-consuming than manual volumetric assessment, but has greater interrater variability.[71]

For distinguishing patients with AD from non-dementia patients the MTA scale reaches around 85% sensitivity and specificity.[72,74] When combined with the Mini Mental State Examination, high sensitivity and specificity of 95% and 98%, respectively, are obtained.[71] MTA also reaches relatively high sensitivity for the diagnosis of other dementias (82%). However, as a consequence, its diagnostic performance in discriminating AD from other dementias is limited. Diagnostic accuracy using volumetric measurements is similar.[71,72,75] However, volumetric imaging allows for serial measurements, which may be more specific than single measurements. As also mentioned in part I, from a meta-analysis including nearly 600 patients with AD and more than 200 healthy controls, the rate of hippocampal atrophy per year was estimated to be more than 3-fold higher in patients than in controls.[20] Atrophy rates in patients with MCI are found to be higher than healthy controls but lower than patients with AD, suggesting a continuum of atrophy rate as a function of disease severity.[20,72]

MTA needs to be rated in both hemispheres separately to assess the presence and degree of

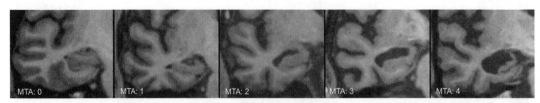

Fig. 19. Coronal T1-weighted images of the hippocampus for stages 0 to 4 of the MTA rating scale (see **Table 3**). Note progressive widening of the choroid fissure (from stage 1 onwards) and temporal horn (from stage 2 onwards), as well as hippocampal body volume loss (stages 3 and 4).

Table 3
Visual rating scale of MTA

	Choroid Fissure	Temporal Horn	Hippocampal Height
MTA = 0	Normal	Normal	Normal
MTA = 1	Widened	Normal	Normal
MTA = 2	Moderately widened	Widened	Reduced
MTA = 3	Severely widened	Moderately widened	Moderately reduced
MTA = 4	Severely widened	Severely widened	Severely reduced

Data from Scheltens P, Leys D, Barkhof F, et al. Atrophy of medial temporal lobes on MRI in "probable" Alzheimer's disease and normal ageing: diagnostic value and neuropsychological correlates. J Neurol Neurosurg Psychiatry 1992;55(10):967–72.

asymmetry. In a meta-analysis of 700 individuals with AD, 365 with MCI and more than 1000 healthy control individuals asymmetrical hippocampal volume was consistently found, with the hippocampus on the left being smaller than on the right. Asymmetry was least in the AD group, being reduced with disease progression.[67] A certain degree of asymmetry of hippocampal volume may thus be expected, especially at earlier stages of the disease. Asymmetry of the hippocampus does therefore not exclude AD, although marked asymmetry suggests an alternative diagnosis, most notably FTD (see article elsewhere in this issue). However, certain atypical presentations of AD are also accompanied by marked asymmetrical atrophy of brain regions including the hippocampus.

Atypical Presentation of AD

Distinctly different patterns of brain atrophy from typical AD may be observed in patients with so-called atypical AD. These are often patients without the APOE ε4 genotype or those presenting younger than 65 years. Atrophy in these patients consists of focal cortical atrophy, which has an estimated relative prevalence of 6% to 14%.[1] Hippocampal atrophy, the hallmark finding in typical AD, is less prominent and may even be absent.

Focal cortical atrophies are associated with the neuropathologic findings of typical AD, but are clinically and radiologically distinct in that a single cognitive domain, not related to memory, is predominantly affected and imaging shows atrophy in the brain region functionally associated to the affected domain. These syndromes include posterior cortical atrophy (PCA) and logopenic progressive aphasia (LPA), both being associated with a posterior pattern of atrophy. Despite more rapid disease progression than in typical AD, longitudinal studies indicate that the pattern of symptoms is relatively stable over time.[64]

Early-onset AD

Early-onset AD is arbitrarily defined as AD with an onset of symptoms before the age of 65 years. Patients have been shown to have greater frontal volume loss, with sparing of the medial temporal area, compared with typical, late-onset AD.[76] The disease progresses faster than late-onset AD, with a higher prevalence of neocortical function impairment. Compared with healthy controls, patients with early-onset AD have greater temporoparietal atrophy.[77] One of the areas that is primarily affected in early-onset AD is the precuneus. In a study of 55 patients Karas and colleagues[78] found disproportionate and independent precuneus atrophy in patients with early-onset compared with late-onset AD, and the relative absence of hippocampal atrophy (**Fig. 20**).

PCA

Patients with PCA have an early and prominent impairment of visual and visuospatial skills, with less prominent memory loss, and show associated atrophy of the parieto-occipital and posterior temporal cortices. Atrophy is generally asymmetrical, the right hemisphere being more affected than the left.[76] In the largest histopathologic series to date of 27 patients, AD pathology was present in 14 (67%).[79] AD-specific biomarkers such as amyloid-specific molecular imaging and CSF protein spectra are frequently found to be positive in patients with clinical and imaging findings of PCA, further supporting the concept of AD as the most likely underlying pathology.[80,81]

Despite the predominance of AD pathology underlying PCA, sometimes coined visual AD,[82] it is undecided whether it should be considered as part of the spectrum of presentations constituting AD or a distinct entity. The syndrome is therefore generally referred to as PCA, independent of the underlying neuropathology, which apart from AD also includes Parkinson disease, DLB, corticobasal degeneration, and prion-associated disease.[64,83] In

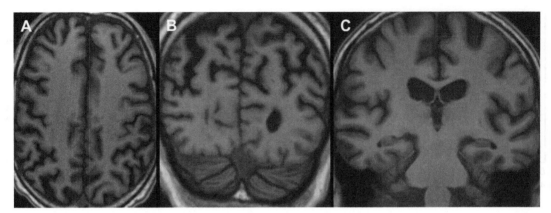

Fig. 20. Sixty-year-old man with early-onset AD. Transverse (*A*) and coronal (*B, C*) T1-weighted images show marked parietal atrophy (*A, B*) without hippocampal atrophy (*C*).

keeping with the commonly underlying AD pathology, most patients eventually progress to a more global and diffuse pattern of cognitive impairment.

LPA

LPA has relatively recently been described as a clinically, neuropathologically, and radiologically distinct subtype of primary progressive aphasia (PPA).[84] The syndrome is characterized by language disorders rather than memory impairment, which consists of slow speech and deficits in sentence repetition. Although speech is slow, it is linguistically still considered fluent because of the lack of grammatical or speech errors. On brain imaging there is marked asymmetrical atrophy of the posterior temporal cortex, including the posterior superior and middle temporal gyri, and the inferior parietal lobule, with the left hemisphere more affected than the right.[76,85] During the course of the disease, atrophy progresses to the posterior cingulate and into the more anterior and medial parts of the temporal lobe, including the hippocampus.[85] However, early in the disease hippocampal volume may be normal. Similar to patients with typical late-onset AD, most patients with LPA have positive AD molecular imaging and CSF biomarkers.[85]

Clinically, LPA is difficult to distinguish from the other PPA subtypes, which have predominantly underlying FTD disease.[86] Structural brain imaging plays an important role in differential diagnosis (see article elsewhere in this issue).

Differential Diagnoses of AD

The most important differential diagnoses of AD, depending on age of onset, are vascular dementia (VaD), FTD (see article elsewhere in this issue), nonfluent and semantic subtypes of PPA, DLB

(see article elsewhere in this issue), and CJD, in which MR imaging typically shows marked hyperintensity on T2-weighted sequences bilaterally in the caudate nucleus and the putamen, and to a lesser extent in the thalamus and neocortex (**Fig. 21**). Diffusion-weighted imaging, showing restricted diffusion in the affected gray matter, seems to be the most sensitive sequence to detect CJD-related abnormalities.[87] Overall sensitivity and specificity are reported to be 60% to 90% and 80% to 95%, respectively.[88,89] VaD is considered separately in the next section, addressing the complex interrelationship of cerebrovascular disease and AD. Especially in the early stages of the disease, when symptoms are often nonspecific, differential diagnosis may be challenging. However, accurate differentiation between the several types of dementia is of especially great relevance in the early stages, when future treatments might have their greatest effect and when most can be gained in terms of symptom reduction and increased quality of life.

Cerebrovascular Disease and AD

In elderly individuals, cerebrovascular disease is the second most common pathology underlying dementia after AD.

VaD

VaD is a heterogeneous entity, including large and small vessel disease, involving the gray or white matter, and which may arise from local or systemic causes.[63] The most common underlying pathology is small vessel disease, leading to diffuse confluent white matter changes (also known as Binswanger disease) and multiple lacunar infarcts of the deep white and (notably the thalamic) gray matter. Confluent WMLs are caused by incomplete infarction of the white matter, leading to demyelination,

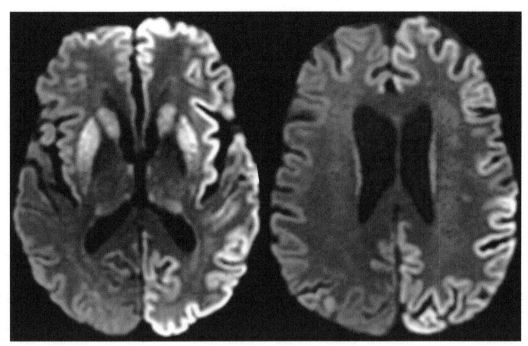

Fig. 21. Sixty-nine-year-old woman with CJD. Transverse diffusion-weighted images show marked hyperintensity of the caudate nucleus and putamen bilaterally, as well as of the neocortex in the left more than the right hemisphere.

edema, gliosis, spongiosis, and breakdown of the ependymal lining.[63] Typically, the subcortical U-fibers are spared. When infarction of the deep perforating arteries is complete, lacunar infarcts occur, which are visualized on MR imaging as small lesions with signal intensity of CSF on all sequences, surrounded by a rim of T2-weighted hyperintensity. A multilacunar state is also known as état lacunaire, not to be confused with état criblé, which is the term used for multiple EPVSs in the basal ganglia, often accompanied by confluent WMLs. Both states are considered pathologic and manifestations of small vessel disease.

Large vessel disease manifests as multiple strategic infarcts, cortical laminar necrosis, or hippocampal necrosis.

Diagnostic criteria for VaD

Because a causative link between cerebrovascular disease and dementia generally cannot be established with certainty, and cerebrovascular changes are common in healthy elderly individuals, as outlined in the first part of this article, there are strict criteria to diagnose VaD set out by the National Institute of Neurologic Disorders and Stroke and Association Internationale pour la Recherche et l'Enseignement en Neurosciences (NINDS-AIREN).[90] A patient must meet the criteria of a dementia syndrome, have

evidence of cerebrovascular disease on clinical examination and on imaging, and there has to be a temporal relationship between the onset of dementia and cerebrovascular disease. Radiological criteria are crucial to diagnosis and specified in detail,[91] requiring both topographic and severity criteria to be met. Confluent WMLs need to involve at least 25% of the total white matter to reach the diagnosis of VaD (see **Fig. 8**). Lacunar infarcts need to involve multiple basal ganglia and the frontal white matter, and thalamic lesions need to be bilateral. Strategic large vessel infarcts meet the criteria when they involve the following territories: bilateral anterior cerebral artery, paramedian thalamic, inferior medial temporal lobe, parietotemporal and temporo-occipital association areas and angular gyrus, superior frontal and parietal watershed areas in the dominant hemisphere.[91,92]

VaD and AD

There seems to be a complex interrelationship between AD and cerebrovascular disease that extends beyond the coexistence of these 2 disease processes. Imaging features of small vessel disease are seen at higher frequency in AD than in healthy controls. Cerebrovascular disease and AD often coexist, whereas stroke often exacerbates preexisting, sometimes previously subclinical,

Table 4
Suggested MR imaging protocol for dementia

	Sequence	Findings
3D	T1-weighted	Atrophy Coronal plane: hippocampal atrophy Sagittal plane: precuneus atrophy
Two-dimensional (2D)/3D	T2-FLAIR	Atrophy, white and gray matter signal abnormalities Coronal plane: hippocampal signal abnormalities
2D transverse	TSE/FSE T2-weighted	White and gray matter signal abnormalities, particularly thalamus and posterior fossa
2D transverse	Diffusion-weighted imaging	Diffusion restriction
2D transverse	T2*-weighted	Microbleeds, subpial hemosiderosis

disease. Furthermore, AD and VaD share common risk factors, such as diabetes and hypertension, as well as genetic factors for brain tissue vulnerability (presenilins, amyloid precursor protein, APOE genes). In patients with MCI, MTA predicts cognitive function better than small vessel disease, although the severity of baseline white matter hyperintensities is a significant predictor of cognitive decline.[93]

Microbleeds, considered to be a manifestation of CAA, are seen at high frequency in patients with AD (see **Figs. 13** and **15**). CAA is a microangiopathy with β-amyloid deposition in the vessel walls. On brain imaging, the presence of 3 or more microbleeds (at 1.5 T) in a lobar distribution is suggestive of CAA,[94] and other features include subpial siderosis and evidence of past lobar hemorrhage. Although sporadic CAA is commonly seen in elderly individuals, being the leading cause of lobar hemorrhage, in its severe form it is also recognized as a risk factor for dementia. This condition typically constitutes a subcortical VaD, but severe CAA is also considered a feature of AD, sharing the APOE ε4 allele as a common risk factor. The fact that AD patients with many microbleeds perform worse on neuropsychological tests and have higher levels of Aβ-1-42 in their CSF has led to the

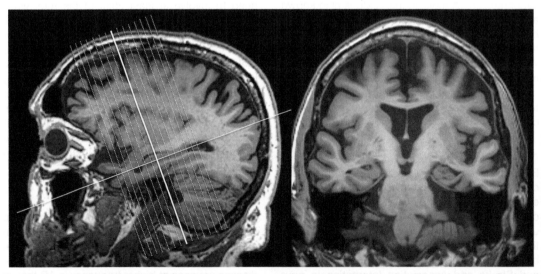

Fig. 22. For optimal assessment of the hippocampus, coronal reconstructions need to be made perpendicular to the plane of the hippocampus. The thin line is aligned along the hippocampus in the sagittal T1-weighted image (*left*), with the thick and dashed lines indicating the plane of coronal reconstruction. Right-hand image shows the resulting coronal section at the level of the thick line.

idea that CAA reflects the combination of AD and vascular damage.[63]

It is not clear how to interpret the interrelationship between vascular disease and AD, whether they happen to coexist in 1 patient, or whether they have a synergistic relationship aggravating each other's effect.

Imaging Protocol and Report in AD

We recommend that the MR imaging scanning protocol includes T1-weighted, T2-weighted, T2-FLAIR, diffusion-weighted, and T2*-weighted sequences (Table 4). Contrast is not indicated routinely, although it is indicated if granulomatous disease, vasculitis, and infection are considered as differential diagnoses.

Three-dimensional (3D) T1-weighted sequences are best suited to assess presence and degree of atrophy and can be reformatted in any plane, including the coronal plane, aligned perpendicular to the plane of the hippocampus, to assess MTA (Fig. 22) and the sagittal plane to assess atrophy of the precuneus in early AD. WMLs are best visualized on a T2-FLAIR sequence, preferably using a 3D sequence, which again allows for the reconstruction in the coronal plane to scrutinize the hippocampus for focal signal abnormalities, and

---

Box 4
Summary of structural MR imaging findings in the (differential) diagnosis of AD

Typical AD
- Disproportionate hippocampal atrophy with temporoparietal atrophy
- Relative sparing of the primary motor and sensory cortex
- Bilateral, more or less symmetric
- Microbleeds in a lobar, subcortical distribution

Atypical AD
- No or little hippocampal atrophy
- Focal cortical atrophy
  - Precuneus: early-onset AD
  - Parieto-occipital and posterior temporal lobe: PCA
  - Posterior temporal cortex and the inferior parietal lobule: LPA
- Marked asymmetry of atrophy
  - Right more than left: PCA
  - Left more than right: LPA

FTD
- Bilateral frontal and temporal atrophy with anterior to posterior gradient
  - Left more than right anterior perisylvian region: NFPA
  - Left more than right ventrolateral temporal region: SD
- (Asymmetrical) hippocampal atrophy, more pronounced anteriorly
- Disproportionate widening of the frontal horns.
- Relative sparing of the parietal and occipital lobes

CJD
- T2-hyperintensity and diffusion restriction bilaterally in the caudate nucleus and putamen, and to a lesser extent in the thalamus and neocortex

DLB
- Medial temporal lobe and GCA
- Relative sparing of the primary motor and sensory cortex
- Less extensive than AD when accounting for disease severity

Abbreviations: NFPA, non-fluent progressive aphasia; SD, semantic dementia.

significantly reduces the CSF flow artifact in the posterior fossa and third ventricle.[95] However, because of reduced sensitivity of FLAIR in the posterior fossa and the diencephalon, specifically the thalamus, a standard T2-weighted sequence also needs to be included.[96] Diffusion-weighted imaging allows for the detection of recent ischemic changes, as well as for visualization of those areas of diffusion restriction characteristic of CJD. T2*-weighted imaging, with low flip angle and long echo time to increase susceptibility sensitivity, is required to detect microbleeds occurring in the context of CAA.

Reporting MR imaging findings in dementia includes both those pointing toward the pathology underlying the dementia syndrome and those suggesting an alternative cause of neurocognitive degeneration. The latter include focal abnormalities such as brain tumor or subdural hematoma. The hippocampus needs to be scrutinized for signal abnormality on T2-weighted sequences to diagnose ischemia or sclerosis. Areas of diffusion restriction may indicate pathology such as acute ischemia, herpes simplex encephalitis, alcoholic encephalopathy, or CJD. T2-weighted hyperintensity in certain brain regions may point to a specific diagnosis, such as in the periaquaductal gray or mammillary bodies in case of alcoholic encephalopathy.

The radiological report further needs to include a structured and standardized assessment of the GCA, the medial temporal lobe and WML load, according to, for instance, the GCA, MTA, and ARWMC visual rating scales, respectively (see **Tables 1–3**). Atrophy should always be rated on the same imaging sequence, preferably the FLAIR or T1-weighted sequence. The degree of asymmetry, as well as focal regions of atrophy, should be reported separately. Both the number and distribution of microbleeds needs to be reported. Large and small vessel cerebrovascular changes need to be specified according to the topographic and severity operational NINDS-AIREN criteria to enable diagnosis of VaD.[91]

A summary of findings (**Box 4**) aids to reach a likely and differential diagnosis of the disease underlying the patient's dementia syndrome.

REFERENCES

1. Dubois B, Feldman HH, Jacova C, et al. Research criteria for the diagnosis of Alzheimer's disease: revising the NINCDS-ADRDA criteria. Lancet Neurol 2007;6(8):734–46.

2. Pelletier D, Garrison K, Henry R. Measurement of whole-brain atrophy in multiple sclerosis. J Neuroimaging 2004;14(Suppl 3):11S–9S.

3. Ashburner J, Friston KJ. Voxel-based morphometry–the methods. Neuroimage 2000;11(6 Pt 1):805–21.

4. de Boer R, Vrooman HA, van der Lijn F, et al. White matter lesion extension to automatic brain tissue segmentation on MRI. Neuroimage 2009;45(4):1151–61.

5. Smith SM, Rao A, De Stefano N, et al. Longitudinal and cross-sectional analysis of atrophy in Alzheimer's disease: cross-validation of BSI, SIENA and SIENAX. Neuroimage 2007;36(4):1200–6.

6. Freeborough PA, Fox NC. The boundary shift integral: an accurate and robust measure of cerebral volume changes from registered repeat MRI. IEEE Trans Med Imaging 1997;16(5):623–9.

7. de Boer R, Vrooman HA, Ikram MA, et al. Accuracy and reproducibility study of automatic MRI brain tissue segmentation methods. Neuroimage 2010; 51(3):1047–56.

8. DeCarli C, Massaro J, Harvey D, et al. Measures of brain morphology and infarction in the framingham heart study: establishing what is normal. Neurobiol Aging 2005;26(4):491–510.

9. Ikram MA, Vrooman HA, Vernooij MW, et al. Brain tissue volumes in the general elderly population. The Rotterdam Scan Study. Neurobiol Aging 2008; 29(6):882–90.

10. Enzinger C, Fazekas F, Matthews PM, et al. Risk factors for progression of brain atrophy in aging: six-year follow-up of normal subjects. Neurology 2005;64(10):1704–11.

11. Allen JS, Bruss J, Brown CK, et al. Normal neuroanatomical variation due to age: the major lobes and a parcellation of the temporal region. Neurobiol Aging 2005;26(9):1245–60 [discussion: 1279–82].

12. Fotenos AF, Snyder AZ, Girton LE, et al. Normative estimates of cross-sectional and longitudinal brain volume decline in aging and AD. Neurology 2005; 64(6):1032–9.

13. Jernigan TL, Archibald SL, Fennema-Notestine C, et al. Effects of age on tissues and regions of the cerebrum and cerebellum. Neurobiol Aging 2001; 22(4):581–94.

14. Liu RS, Lemieux L, Bell GS, et al. A longitudinal study of brain morphometrics using quantitative magnetic resonance imaging and difference image analysis. Neuroimage 2003;20(1):22–33.

15. Schmidt R, Ropele S, Enzinger C, et al. White matter lesion progression, brain atrophy, and cognitive decline: the Austrian stroke prevention study. Ann Neurol 2005;58(4):610–6.

16. Konrad C, Ukas T, Nebel C, et al. Defining the human hippocampus in cerebral magnetic resonance images–an overview of current segmentation protocols. Neuroimage 2009;47(4):1185–95.

17. van der Lijn F, den Heijer T, Breteler MM, et al. Hippocampus segmentation in MR images using atlas registration, voxel classification, and graph cuts. Neuroimage 2008;43(4):708–20.

18. Leung KK, Barnes J, Ridgway GR, et al. Automated cross-sectional and longitudinal hippocampal volume measurement in mild cognitive impairment and Alzheimer's disease. Neuroimage 2010;51(4):1345–59.

19. den Heijer T, van der Lijn F, Koudstaal PJ, et al. A 10-year follow-up of hippocampal volume on magnetic resonance imaging in early dementia and cognitive decline. Brain 2010;133(Pt 4):1163–72.

20. Barnes J, Bartlett JW, Van De Pol LA, et al. A meta-analysis of hippocampal atrophy rates in Alzheimer's disease. Neurobiol Aging 2009;30(11):1711–23.

21. Fazekas F, Chawluk JB, Alavi A, et al. MR signal abnormalities at 1.5 T in Alzheimer's dementia and normal aging. AJR Am J Roentgenol 1987;149(2):351–6.

22. Wahlund LO, Barkhof F, Fazekas F, et al. A new rating scale for age-related white matter changes applicable to MRI and CT. Stroke 2001;32(6):1318–22.

23. Scheltens P, Barkhof F, Leys D, et al. A semiquantative rating scale for the assessment of signal hyperintensities on magnetic resonance imaging. J Neurol Sci 1993;114(1):7–12.

24. Kapeller P, Barber R, Vermeulen RJ, et al. Visual rating of age-related white matter changes on magnetic resonance imaging: scale comparison, interrater agreement, and correlations with quantitative measurements. Stroke 2003;34(2):441–5.

25. Mantyla R, Erkinjuntti T, Salonen O, et al. Variable agreement between visual rating scales for white matter hyperintensities on MRI. Comparison of 13 rating scales in a poststroke cohort. Stroke 1997;28(8):1614–23.

26. Pantoni L, Garcia JH. Pathogenesis of leukoaraiosis: a review. Stroke 1997;28(3):652–9.

27. Patel B, Markus HS. Magnetic resonance imaging in cerebral small vessel disease and its use as a surrogate disease marker. Int J Stroke 2011;6(1):47–59.

28. Debette S, Markus HS. The clinical importance of white matter hyperintensities on brain magnetic resonance imaging: systematic review and meta-analysis. BMJ 2010;341:c3666.

29. Barkhof F, van Walderveen M. Characterization of tissue damage in multiple sclerosis by nuclear magnetic resonance. Philos Trans R Soc Lond B Biol Sci 1999;354(1390):1675–86.

30. Basser PJ, Jones DK. Diffusion-tensor MRI: theory, experimental design and data analysis–a technical review. NMR Biomed 2002;15(7–8):456–67.

31. Salat DH, Tuch DS, Greve DN, et al. Age-related alterations in white matter microstructure measured by diffusion tensor imaging. Neurobiol Aging 2005;26(8):1215–27.

32. Sullivan EV, Pfefferbaum A. Diffusion tensor imaging and aging. Neurosci Biobehav Rev 2006;30(6):749–61.

33. Vernooij MW, de Groot M, van der Lugt A, et al. White matter atrophy and lesion formation explain the loss of structural integrity of white matter in aging. Neuroimage 2008;43(3):470–7.

34. Vernooij MW, Ikram MA, Vrooman HA, et al. White matter microstructural integrity and cognitive function in a general elderly population. Arch Gen Psychiatry 2009;66(5):545–53.

35. Charlton RA, Barrick TR, McIntyre DJ, et al. White matter damage on diffusion tensor imaging correlates with age-related cognitive decline. Neurology 2006;66(2):217–22.

36. O'Sullivan M, Jones DK, Summers PE, et al. Evidence for cortical "disconnection" as a mechanism of age-related cognitive decline. Neurology 2001;57(4):632–8.

37. Offenbacher H, Fazekas F, Schmidt R, et al. MR of cerebral abnormalities concomitant with primary intracerebral hematomas. AJNR Am J Neuroradiol 1996;17(3):573–8.

38. Scheid R, Ott DV, Roth H, et al. Comparative magnetic resonance imaging at 1.5 and 3 Tesla for the evaluation of traumatic microbleeds. J Neurotrauma 2007;24(12):1811–6.

39. Vernooij MW, Ikram MA, Wielopolski PA, et al. Cerebral microbleeds: accelerated 3D T2*-weighted GRE MR imaging versus conventional 2D T2*-weighted GRE MR imaging for detection. Radiology 2008;248(1):272–7.

40. Sehgal V, Delproposto Z, Haacke EM, et al. Clinical applications of neuroimaging with susceptibility-weighted imaging. J Magn Reson Imaging 2005;22(4):439–50.

41. Vernooij MW, van der Lugt A, Ikram MA, et al. Prevalence and risk factors of cerebral microbleeds: the Rotterdam Scan Study. Neurology 2008;70(14):1208–14.

42. Poels MM, Vernooij MW, Ikram MA, et al. Prevalence and risk factors of cerebral microbleeds: an update of the Rotterdam scan study. Stroke 2010;41(Suppl 10):S103–6.

43. Mesker DJ, Poels MM, Ikram MA, et al. Lobar distribution of cerebral microbleeds: the Rotterdam Scan Study. Arch Neurol 2011;68(5):656–9.

44. Qiu C, Cotch MF, Sigurdsson S, et al. Cerebral microbleeds, retinopathy, and dementia: the AGES-Reykjavik Study. Neurology 2010;75(24):2221–8.

45. Poels MM, Ikram MA, Van der Lugt A, et al. Cerebral microbleeds are associated with worse cognitive function. The Rotterdam Scan Study. Neurology, in press.

46. Goos JD, Kester MI, Barkhof F, et al. Patients with Alzheimer disease with multiple microbleeds: relation with cerebrospinal fluid biomarkers and cognition. Stroke 2009;40(11):3455–60.

47. Poels MM, Ikram MA, van der Lugt A, et al. Incidence of cerebral microbleeds in the general

population: the Rotterdam Scan Study. Stroke 2011; 42(3):656–61.

48. Goos JD, Henneman WJ, Sluimer JD, et al. Incidence of cerebral microbleeds: a longitudinal study in a memory clinic population. Neurology 2010; 74(24):1954–60.

49. Vermeer SE, Longstreth WT Jr, Koudstaal PJ. Silent brain infarcts: a systematic review. Lancet Neurol 2007;6(7):611–9.

50. Zhu YC, Dufouil C, Tzourio C, et al. Silent brain infarcts: a review of MRI diagnostic criteria. Stroke 2011;42(4):1140–5.

51. Shima H, Ishimura E, Naganuma T, et al. Decreased kidney function is a significant factor associated with silent cerebral infarction and periventricular hyperintensities. Kidney Blood Press Res 2011;34(6): 430–8.

52. Cheung N, Mosley T, Islam A, et al. Retinal microvascular abnormalities and subclinical magnetic resonance imaging brain infarct: a prospective study. Brain 2010;133(Pt 7):1987–93.

53. Groeschel S, Chong WK, Surtees R, et al. Virchow-Robin spaces on magnetic resonance images: normative data, their dilatation, and a review of the literature. Neuroradiology 2006;48(10):745–54.

54. Zhu YC, Tzourio C, Soumare A, et al. Severity of dilated Virchow-Robin spaces is associated with age, blood pressure, and MRI markers of small vessel disease: a population-based study. Stroke 2010;41(11):2483–90.

55. Doubal FN, MacLullich AM, Ferguson KJ, et al. Enlarged perivascular spaces on MRI are a feature of cerebral small vessel disease. Stroke 2010; 41(3):450–4.

56. Maclullich AM, Wardlaw JM, Ferguson KJ, et al. Enlarged perivascular spaces are associated with cognitive function in healthy elderly men. J Neurol Neurosurg Psychiatry 2004;75(11):1519–23.

57. Zhu YC, Dufouil C, Soumare A, et al. High degree of dilated Virchow-Robin spaces on MRI is associated with increased risk of dementia. J Alzheimers Dis 2010;22(2):663–72.

58. Zhu YC, Dufouil C, Mazoyer B, et al. Frequency and location of dilated Virchow-Robin spaces in elderly people: a population-based 3D MR imaging study. AJNR Am J Neuroradiol 2011;32(4):709–13.

59. Bastos-Leite AJ, van Waesberghe JH, Oen AL, et al. Hippocampal sulcus width and cavities: comparison between patients with Alzheimer disease and non-demented elderly subjects. AJNR Am J Neuroradiol 2006;27(10):2141–5.

60. McKhann G, Drachman D, Folstein M, et al. Clinical diagnosis of Alzheimer's disease: report of the NINCDS-ADRDA Work Group under the auspices of Department of Health and Human Services Task Force on Alzheimer's Disease. Neurology 1984;34(7): 939–44.

61. McKhann GM, Knopman DS, Chertkow H, et al. The diagnosis of dementia due to Alzheimer's disease: recommendations from the National Institute on Aging-Alzheimer's Association workgroups on diagnostic guidelines for Alzheimer's disease. Alzheimers Dement 2011;7:263–9.

62. Braak H, Braak E. Neuropathological stageing of Alzheimer-related changes. Acta Neuropathol 1991;82(4):239–59.

63. Barkhof F, Fox N, Bastos Leite AJ, et al. Neuroimaging in dementia. Berlin, Heidelberg (Germany): Springer-Verlag; 2011.

64. Kramer JH, Miller BL. Alzheimer's disease and its focal variants. Semin Neurol 2000;20(4):447–54.

65. Laakso MP, Soininen H, Partanen K, et al. MRI of the hippocampus in Alzheimer's disease: sensitivity, specificity, and analysis of the incorrectly classified subjects. Neurobiol Aging 1998;19(1):23–31.

66. Du AT, Schuff N, Amend D, et al. Magnetic resonance imaging of the entorhinal cortex and hippocampus in mild cognitive impairment and Alzheimer's disease. J Neurol Neurosurg Psychiatry 2001;71(4):441–7.

67. Shi F, Liu B, Zhou Y, et al. Hippocampal volume and asymmetry in mild cognitive impairment and Alzheimer's disease: meta-analyses of MRI studies. Hippocampus 2009;19(11):1055–64.

68. Achterberg HC, van der Lijn F, den Heijer T, et al. Prediction of dementia by hippocampal shape analysis. In: Wang F, Yan P, Suzuki K, et al, editors. Machine learning in medical imaging. 1st edition. Beijing (China): Springer; 2010. p. 42–9.

69. Costafreda SG, Dinov ID, Tu Z, et al. Automated hippocampal shape analysis predicts the onset of dementia in mild cognitive impairment. Neuroimage 2011;56(1):212–9.

70. Scheltens P, Leys D, Barkhof F, et al. Atrophy of medial temporal lobes on MRI in "probable" Alzheimer's disease and normal ageing: diagnostic value and neuropsychological correlates. J Neurol Neurosurg Psychiatry 1992;55(10):967–72.

71. Wahlund LO, Julin P, Johansson SE, et al. Visual rating and volumetry of the medial temporal lobe on magnetic resonance imaging in dementia: a comparative study. J Neurol Neurosurg Psychiatry 2000;69(5):630–5.

72. Petrella JR, Coleman RE, Doraiswamy PM. Neuroimaging and early diagnosis of Alzheimer disease: a look to the future. Radiology 2003;226(2):315–36.

73. Scheltens P, Launer LJ, Barkhof F, et al. Visual assessment of medial temporal lobe atrophy on magnetic resonance imaging: interobserver reliability. J Neurol 1995;242(9):557–60.

74. Scheltens P, Fox N, Barkhof F, et al. Structural magnetic resonance imaging in the practical assessment of dementia: beyond exclusion. Lancet Neurol 2002;1(1):13–21.

75. Wahlund L-O, Almkvist O, Blennow K, et al. Evidence-based evaluation of magnetic resonance imaging as a diagnostic tool in dementia workup. Top Magn Reson Imaging 2005;16(6):427–37.

76. Migliaccio R, Agosta F, Rascovsky K, et al. Clinical syndromes associated with posterior atrophy: early age at onset AD spectrum. Neurology 2009;73(19): 1571–8.

77. Frisoni GB, Testa C, Sabattoli F, et al. Structural correlates of early and late onset Alzheimer's disease: voxel based morphometric study. J Neurol Neurosurg Psychiatry 2005;76(1):112–4.

78. Karas G, Scheltens P, Rombouts S, et al. Precuneus atrophy in early-onset Alzheimer's disease: a morphometric structural MRI study. Neuroradiology 2007;49(12):967–76.

79. Renner JA, Burns JM, Hou CE, et al. Progressive posterior cortical dysfunction: a clinicopathologic series. Neurology 2004;63(7):1175–80.

80. Seguin J, Formaglio M, Perret-Liaudet A, et al. CSF biomarkers in posterior cortical atrophy. Neurology 2011;76(21):1782–8.

81. Tenovuo O, Kemppainen N, Aalto S, et al. Posterior cortical atrophy: a rare form of dementia with in vivo evidence of amyloid-beta accumulation. J Alzheimers Dis 2008;15(3):351–5.

82. Goethals M, Santens P. Posterior cortical atrophy. Two case reports and a review of the literature. Clin Neurol Neurosurg 2001;103(2):115–9.

83. Caine D. Posterior cortical atrophy: a review of the literature. Neurocase 2004;10(5):382–5.

84. Gorno-Tempini ML, Dronkers NF, Rankin KP, et al. Cognition and anatomy in three variants of primary progressive aphasia. Ann Neurol 2004;55(3): 335–46.

85. Henry ML, Gorno-Tempini ML. The logopenic variant of primary progressive aphasia. Curr Opin Neurol 2010;23(6):633–7.

86. Bonner MF, Ash S, Grossman M. The new classification of primary progressive aphasia into semantic, logopenic, or nonfluent/agrammatic variants. Curr Neurol Neurosci Rep 2010;10(6):484–90.

87. Young GS, Geschwind MD, Fischbein NJ, et al. Diffusion-weighted and fluid-attenuated inversion recovery imaging in Creutzfeldt-Jakob disease: high sensitivity and specificity for diagnosis. AJNR Am J Neuroradiol 2005;26(6):1551–62.

88. Tschampa HJ, Kallenberg K, Urbach H, et al. MRI in the diagnosis of sporadic Creutzfeldt-Jakob disease: a study on inter-observer agreement. Brain 2005;128(Pt 9):2026–33.

89. Schröter A, Zerr I, Henkel K, et al. Magnetic resonance imaging in the clinical diagnosis of Creutzfeldt-Jakob disease. Arch Neurol 2000;57(12):1751–7.

90. Román GC, Tatemichi TK, Erkinjuntti T, et al. Vascular dementia: diagnostic criteria for research studies. Report of the NINDS-AIREN International Workshop. Neurology 1993;43(2):250–60.

91. van Straaten EC, Scheltens P, Knol DL, et al. Operational definitions for the NINDS-AIREN criteria for vascular dementia: an interobserver study. Stroke 2003;34(8):1907–12.

92. van Straaten EC, Scheltens P, Barkhof F. MRI and CT in the diagnosis of vascular dementia. J Neurol Sci 2004;226(1–2):9–12.

93. Small GW, Bookheimer SY, Thompson PM, et al. Current and future uses of neuroimaging for cognitively impaired patients. Lancet Neurol 2008;7(2): 161–72.

94. Knudsen KA, Rosand J, Karluk D, et al. Clinical diagnosis of cerebral amyloid angiopathy: validation of the Boston criteria. Neurology 2001;56(4): 537–9.

95. Rumboldt Z, Marotti M. Magnetization transfer, HASTE, and FLAIR imaging. Magn Reson Imaging Clin N Am 2003;11(3):471–92.

96. Bastos Leite AJ, van Straaten EC, Scheltens P, et al. Thalamic lesions in vascular dementia: low sensitivity of fluid-attenuated inversion recovery (FLAIR) imaging. Stroke 2004;35(2):415–9.

Molecular Neuroimaging in Alzheimer's Disease

Hiroshi Matsuda, MD, PhD*, Etsuko Imabayashi, MD, PhD

KEYWORDS

- PET • PiB • Alzheimer's disease
- Mild cognitive impairment

Dementia is a serious loss of cognitive ability in a previously unimpaired person beyond what might be expected from normal aging. Dementia that begins gradually and worsens progressively over several years is usually caused by neurodegenerative disease, that is, by conditions affecting only or primarily the neurons of the brain and causing gradual but irreversible loss of function of these cells. Worldwide increases in the number of people with dementia, the highest proportion of whom are affected by Alzheimer's disease (AD), have made its early diagnosis a major research and clinical priority. The cause of AD is unknown, but typical changes in the brain are neuronal loss, numerous globs of sticky proteins (β-amyloid [Aβ] plaques) in the spaces between neurons, a tangled bundle of fibrils within neurons (neurofibrillary tangles). Although it is still unclear what the relationship is between amyloid pathology and neuronal degeneration, progressive neuronal loss, and subsequent atrophy of various cortical gray matter structures, the most prominent hypothesis[1] for the cause of AD remains the amyloid cascade hypothesis, which holds that the Aβ peptide is the key to the initiation and progression of the disease. Pathologic studies are insufficient to validate this theory, because they are always inevitably cross-sectional and cannot determine how key events are temporally related to each other. During the past several years, amyloid imaging has established itself alongside magnetic resonance (MR) imaging and fluorodeoxyglucose (FDG)-positron emission tomography (PET) as a surrogate marker for the investigation of brain aging and dementia.

Functional neuroimaging, such as FDG-PET and brain perfusion single-photon emission computed tomography (SPECT), has been widely used for imaging biomarkers of AD. Recent advances in instruments have facilitated investigations of functional alterations in fine structures of not only cortical but also subcortical areas with high spatial resolution. Metabolic and perfusion reductions in the parietotemporal association cortex are recognized as a diagnostic pattern for AD. Outstanding progress in the diagnostic accuracy of these modalities has been achieved using statistical analysis on a voxel-by-voxel basis after anatomic standardization of individual scans to a standardized brain volume template instead of visual inspection or a volume-of-interest technique. In a very early stage of AD, this statistical approach revealed hypometabolism or hypoperfusion in the posterior cingulate cortex and precuneus. In some countries where FDG-PET has not yet been accepted for reimbursement for the detection of dementia in the health insurance system, more widely available brain perfusion SPECT has been used for the imaging diagnosis of AD. FDG-PET is superior to SPECT in diagnosing early AD because of its higher sensitivity and higher spatial resolution, and FDG-PET offers many advantages for detecting abnormalities in the AD brain. SPECT

This work was supported by a grant from the Grant-in-Aid for Scientific Research (C), Ministry of Education, Culture, Sports, Science and Technology, Japan (21591578).

The authors have nothing to disclose.

Department of Nuclear Medicine, Saitama Medical University International Medical Center, 1397-1, Yamane, Hidaka, Saitama, 350-1298, Japan

* Corresponding author.

E-mail address: matsudah@saitama-med.ac.jp

offers the advantages of lower cost and ease of access, which could lead to a large increase in the number of cases studied using this technique. Although FDG-PET shows more robust separation of patients with AD from healthy volunteers than SPECT, good correspondence of changes in the parietotemporal and posterior cingulate cortices and precuneus in mild to moderate AD is observed using voxel-based statistical image analysis between FDG-PET and SPECT.

Amyloid imaging allows for more rigorous quantification of the distribution and burden of amyloid, and enables direct comparison of these measures with simultaneously derived cognitive metrics in contrast to the significant delay between behavioral assessment and autopsy often seen in postmortem studies.

Among several compounds that have been developed for the imaging of amyloid, N-methyl-[11C]2-(4′-methyl-aminophenyl)-6-hydroxybezothiazole or simply Pittsburgh compound-B (PiB)[2] is a derivative of the amyloid-binding dye thioflavin T and the most extensively validated tracer. It binds to aggregated, fibrillar Aβ deposits, such as those found in the cerebral cortex and striatum, but not to the amorphous Aβ deposits, such as those that predominate in the cerebellum. The first PiB-PET study in humans[3] was performed in patients with mild AD, in whom the uptake pattern was consistent with Aβ plaque deposition described in postmortem studies of AD brains. Postmortem studies of patients who showed increased PiB deposition during life showed high correlations between in vivo PiB accumulation and in vitro measures of Aβ pathology.[4,5] This article reviews the rapidly expanding literature applying PiB-PET to study cognitively normal volunteers and patients with mild cognitive impairment

(MCI) and AD and summarizes the contribution of PiB-PET in understanding the association between amyloid plaques, aging, and dementia.

PiB-PET IMAGE ANALYSIS

Although visual reading of PiB images seems more accurate than that of FDG for identification of AD, better accuracy is obtained using a quantitative approach without requiring the expertise of readers.[6] PiB binding to Aβ plaque in the gray matter is specific and reversible, whereas PiB binding in the white matter is nonspecific and nonsaturable.[7] The relatively slow kinetics of PiB makes the specific PiB uptake in the gray matter prominent at later time points, which may impede the quantification of Aβ deposits because of the short half-life of ^{11}C-labeled tracer. To overcome this drawback in quantification, three-dimensional dynamic sampling of emission data for the whole brain is desirable, lasting 70 to 90 minutes after tracer injection. Application of the linear models developed by Logan[8] to these sampling data has become a standard calculation method for robust quantification in PiB studies (Fig. 1). Logan analysis is used to calculate the distribution volume of ligand tracers that have reversible binding kinetics. The choice of cerebellar cortex as a reference region that has no specific PiB deposition enables calculation of a distribution volume ratio (DVR) without arterial plasma data sampling as a slope of a graphical plot.[9] The DVR equals binding potential + 1. The pons can also be chosen as a reference area.[10] On the other hand, the standardized uptake value ratio (SUVR) has been proposed as a more feasible semiquantitative analysis than DVR (Fig. 2).[11] SUVR is calculated by computing the

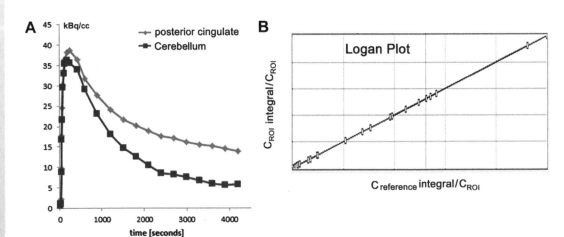

Fig. 1. Typical time-activity curves from dynamic PiB-PET studies from a patient with AD (A) and graphical analysis using a Logan plot (B). Using cerebellar cortex as input, the DVR in the posterior cingulate cortex is determined as a slope of a graphical plot without arterial plasma data sampling.

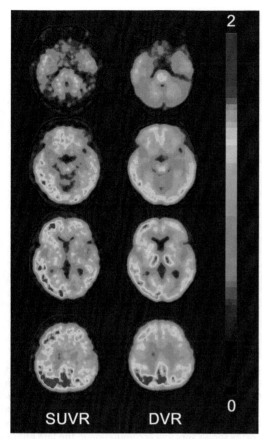

Fig. 2. Comparison of SUVR and DVR images. DVR provides better image quality than SUVR. A longer period of approximately 70 minutes is required for data acquisition for DVR compared with 20 minutes for SUVR.

region/cerebellum ratio at later time points. The optimal time range was studied by McNamee and colleagues[12]; their suggestion was to use a 40- to 60-minute period in studies limited by low injected dose, or a 50- to 70-minute period because of greater measurement stability, especially for longitudinal multisite studies (**Fig. 3**). The advantages of the SUVR approach are large effect sizes for AD and control group differences, and the possibility of obtaining the required data from a single short scan of 20 minutes. The disadvantages of this approach are the lower test-retest variability compared with the DVR approach and the potential for time-varying outcomes.[11] It also has the inherent bias of a tendency to overestimate PiB deposition.[12] The use of a standardized volume-of-interest template with spatially normalized PiB images to the same standardized space has been proposed as an automated voxel-based method for PiB deposition analysis.[13]

Regions that share a border with lower-binding or higher-binding structures are susceptible to partial volume effects because of a blurring caused by the low resolution of PET. Because gray matter, white matter, and cerebrospinal fluid (CSF) have different PiB uptake patterns, all gray matter boarders undergo partial volume effects. Atrophy of a region that increases the amount of neighboring CSF accentuates these partial volume effects. Applying partial volume correction to PiB-PET has been expected to increase the PiB deposition in atrophied gray matter and lead to more accurate quantification.[13,14] Partial volume correction is usually performed using segmented gray matter from three-dimensional MR imaging coregistered to PiB images.

PiB-PET IN NORMAL CONTROLS

Several autopsy studies have reported that significant Aβ deposits can be found post mortem in more than 30% of cognitively normal older individuals and that the extent of Aβ pathology may be indistinguishable from that found in AD.[15,16] In accordance with these autopsy results, several PiB-PET studies have consistently detected increased PiB binding in a subset of normal older volunteers (**Fig. 4**), with the proportion of PiB-positive cases ranging from 10% to 30% depending on the age of the cohort and the threshold for defining PiB positivity.[9,14,17–20] In contrast, increased binding has not been reported in young normal controls. Several studies suggest preferential PiB deposition in the prefrontal cortex and posterior cingulate/precuneus similar to the regions of earliest Aβ deposition noted in autopsy studies.[21] Some older controls show a distribution pattern of PiB binding that is essentially indistinguishable from that seen in AD. The high rate of PiB positivity in normal controls suggests that a positive PiB scan cannot be interpreted without a careful clinical evaluation and emphasizes that amyloid imaging alone must not serve as a surrogate for a clinical diagnosis of AD.

The most important risk factors for AD are age, family history, and heredity. The relationship between these risk factors and PiB deposition has been investigated using a voxel-based statistical analysis. Advancing age increases PiB-positive frequency in normal controls: 18% in those aged 60 to 69 years, rising to 65% in those older than 80 years.[22] The prevalence of Aβ deposition, as detected post mortem in cognitively normal subjects, exponentially increases with advancing age. The prevalence of PiB-positive normal controls increases with advancing age in a similar exponential fashion but precedes the postmortem study by 10 to 15 years. Aβ deposition seems almost inevitable with advancing age.

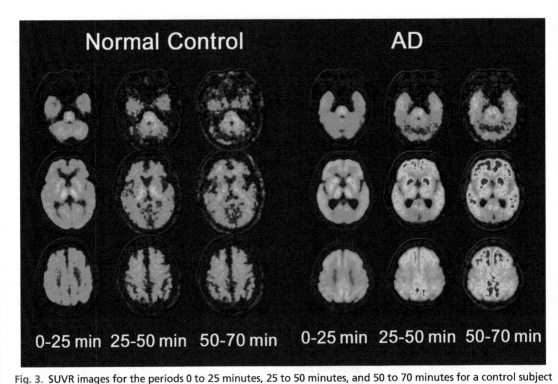

Fig. 3. SUVR images for the periods 0 to 25 minutes, 25 to 50 minutes, and 50 to 70 minutes for a control subject and a patient with AD. Note temporal changes in PiB distribution. The main factors determining PiB distribution changed from perfusion in an early phase to deposition in Aβ in a late phase. A control individual shows no accumulation in cerebral cortex but nonspecific accumulation in white matter in the late phase (PiB-negative). A patient with AD shows prominent PiB accumulation in the entire cerebral cortex except for occipital cortex and striatum in the late phase (PiB-positive). The cerebellar cortex shows very low accumulation in the late phase.

A recent study shows that normal controls with a parent affected by late-onset AD have increased PiB deposition in brain regions typically affected in patients with clinical AD compared with normal controls with no family history. In addition, significant parent-of-origin effects on Aβ deposition were found.[23] Normal controls with mothers affected by late-onset AD show increased and more widespread PiB deposition than those with affected fathers. Another recent study showed that PiB deposition in normal controls correlates with apolipoprotein E (APOE) ε4 gene dose, which is the best known genetic risk factor for AD.[24] The APOE4 allele increases the risk of the disease by 3 times in heterozygous individuals and 15 times in homozygotes. Emerging evidence suggests there may be other risk factors for AD. Epidemiologic studies suggest that cardiovascular risk factors such as increased blood pressure in midlife are associated with increased risk of AD in late life. Langbaum and colleagues[25] revealed that systolic blood pressure and pulse pressure were both positively correlated with PiB depositions. These preliminary findings provide additional evidence that higher BP, which is likely to reflect arterial stiffness during late midlife, may be associated with

increased risk of presymptomatic AD. There is some evidence[26] that only angiotensin receptor blockers and angiotensin-converting enzyme inhibitors, and not other blood-pressure–lowering medications, are associated with reduced risk of AD. Antihypertensive treatments may protect against AD neuropathology, potentially by reducing vascular and arterial stiffness, thereby increasing blood flow to the brain and aiding in the removal of Aβ.

A major unresolved issue in AD research is whether cognitively normal people with amyloid deposition are on a trajectory toward AD, or whether the disease is benign in these individuals. Cross-sectional studies evaluating the influence of PiB binding on brain structure and cognition in older control individuals have yielded seemingly conflicting results. When individuals are dichotomized into PiB-positive and PiB-negative groups, most studies[9,18,19,27] have not found significant differences in cognitive performance, with the exception of a study[17] that found lower episodic memory scores in the PiB-positive group. In contrast, most studies that evaluated PiB deposition as a continuous variable have found significant negative correlations between PiB uptake and episodic memory

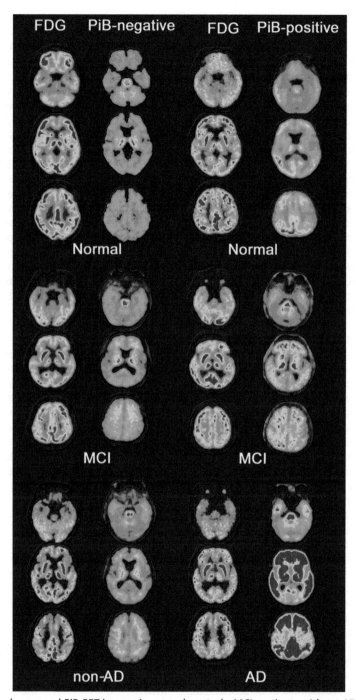

FDG   PiB-negative   FDG   PiB-positive

Normal   Normal

MCI   MCI

non-AD   AD

Fig. 4. Fluorodeoxyglucose and PiB-PET images in normal controls, MCI, patients without AD, and patients with AD. Both PiB-negative and PiB-positive findings are shown in normal controls and patients with MCI. PiB is useful for differentiating patients with and without AD.

scores. Mormino and colleagues[20] revealed significant correlations between PiB deposition and episodic memory, PiB deposition and hippocampal volume, as well as hippocampal volume and episodic memory. This observation suggests that declining episodic memory in older individuals may be caused by Aβ-induced hippocampal atrophy. Becker and colleagues[28] found the significant Aβ-associated cortical thinning particularly in parietal and posterior cingulate regions extending into the precuneus in a pattern consistent with early AD among nondemented older individuals. This finding suggests that Aβ-associated neurodegeneration is manifest as cortical thinning in regions vulnerable to early Aβ deposition. Oh and colleagues[29] found that gray matter volume in the left inferior frontal cortex was negatively associated with amyloid deposition across all participants of nondemented older controls, whereas reduced gray matter volume was shown in the posterior cingulate among older controls with high amyloid deposition. This reduction of gray matter volume in the left inferior frontal cortex was associated with poorer working memory performance. The pattern of Aβ deposition as detected by PiB-PET shows substantial spatial overlap with the default mode network comprising a group of brain regions that typically deactivate during externally driven cognitive tasks.[30] Functional connectivity in the default mode network is altered with increasing levels of PiB uptake. These findings highlight structural and cognitive changes in association with the level of Aβ deposition in cognitively intact normal elderly individuals.

Longitudinal studies evaluating the relationship between PiB deposition and cognitive decline or brain atrophy have also yielded conflicting results. Dricoll and colleagues[31] examined associations between PiB deposition and brain volume changes in the preceding years in 57 nondemented individuals. Despite significant longitudinal decline in the volumes of all the regions investigated, no associations were detected between PiB deposition and regional brain volume decline trajectories in the preceding year, nor did the regional volume trajectories differ between those with highest and lowest Aβ burden. These findings suggest that Aβ load does not seem to affect brain volume changes in individuals without dementia. These investigators' observations are in agreement with existing reports on PiB deposition and brain volume loss. Jack and colleagues[32] investigated MR imaging and PiB studies at 2 time points, approximately 1 year apart, to gain insight into the sequence of pathologic events in AD. These investigators reported a dissociation between the rate of amyloid deposition and the rate of neurodegeneration late in life over 1 year of follow-up. Amyloid deposition proceeded at a constant low rate irrespective of clinical status, whereas neurodegeneration accelerated in association with clinical symptoms. These findings suggest that in nondemented elderly individuals, amyloid accumulation does not affect the rate of brain atrophy beyond that already observed as a part of the normal aging process. On the contrary, Villemagne and colleagues[14] reported that normal controls who progressed to MCI or AD over 38 months had significantly lower memory scores, higher baseline, and greater increase of PiB

deposition than those normal controls who did not progress. Sojkova and colleagues[33] also found that longitudinal increases in Aβ deposition varied among individuals. This variability in the annual rate of change was affected by PiB deposition at the initial PET study, and increases were greater in nondemented older adults with an increased Aβ level compared with a minimal Aβ level at the initial evaluation. Furthermore a longitudinal cohort study[34] was performed to determine whether preclinical AD, as detected by PiB-PET in cognitively normal older adults, is associated with a risk of symptomatic AD. Twenty-three of 159 participants with a clinical dementia rating (CDR) of 0 progressed to CDR 0.5 at follow-up assessment. More increased PiB deposition highly predicted progression to CDR 0.5, with a hazard ratio of 4.85. These findings suggest that PiB deposition is not benign, because it is associated with progression to symptomatic AD.

PiB-PET IN MCI

Amyloid imaging can potentially identify patients with MCI who already show Aβ aggregation and are thus in the early clinical phase of AD, and separate them from patients with alternative causes for their cognitive impairment. Dividing patients with MCI into more biologically homogeneous groups may also facilitate their inclusion in clinical trials for AD-specific therapies, allowing these treatments to be tested in patients earlier in the disease course. Perhaps the correct use of antiamyloid monotherapies will be as a prophylactic given long before the onset of symptoms in people at risk of AD.[35]

Numerous studies in MCI have reported that PiB uptake is intermediate between AD and controls (see Fig. 4). However, PiB binding levels in MCI in most studies are bimodal, with most cases showing an AD-like uptake level, a few showing low control-level binding, and a few falling in the intermediate range. Overall, 52% to 87% of patients with MCI show increased PiB binding, depending on the criteria used to diagnose MCI and the threshold used to define PiB positivity.[11,14,17,18,20,27,36–38] Individuals meeting the criteria for amnestic MCI were more likely to be PiB positive than patients with nonamnestic MCI. Villemagner and colleagues[14] reported that progression of MCI to AD occurred in 67% of cases of MCI with high PiB deposition versus 5% of those with low PiB. Forsberg and colleagues[37] reported that 33% (7 of 21) of patients with MCI with increased PiB binding later at clinical follow-up converted to AD. Irrespective of MCI subtypes, longitudinal follow-ups reported that 5 of 13

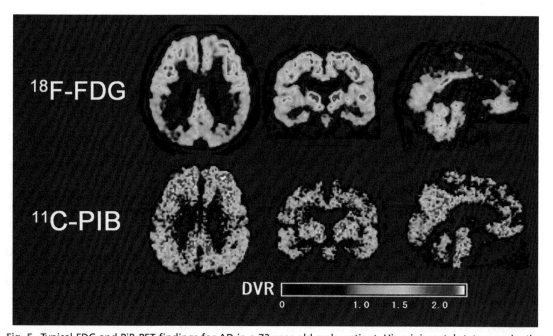

Fig. 5. Typical FDG and PiB-PET findings for AD in a 72-year-old male patient. His minimental state examination score was 18. Note high PiB deposition in the prefrontal cortex and posterior cingulate/precuneus, whereas FDG-PET showed decreased glucose metabolism in posterior cingulate/precuneus and bilateral parietal cortex.

amyloid-positive patients, but 0 of 10 amyloid-negative patients, converted to clinical AD.[38]

PiB-PET IN AD

The initial objective of amyloid imaging with PiB-PET focused on detecting Aβ amyloidosis in patients clinically diagnosed with AD. As expected, most patients with AD show increased PiB deposition (**Fig. 5**).[3,6,9,18,27,39] Using clinical diagnosis as a gold standard, the sensitivity of PiB-PET for AD has been reported as 80% to 100%, with most studies reporting sensitivities of 90% or greater. The significance of a negative PiB scan in a patient clinically diagnosed with AD is not yet clear because of the lack of postmortem data. The proportion of PiB-negative scans in AD is similar to the fraction of patients clinically diagnosed with AD at dementia referral centers who are subsequently found to have an alternative pathology at autopsy,[40] suggesting that many PiB-negative scans in AD may represent a true-negative. A pathology-confirmed false-negative PiB result has been reported,[41] involving a patient with Aβ plaques on frontal brain biopsy who showed low PiB binding when studied with PET 20 months later. Cairns and colleagues[42] reported a PiB-negative patient with reduced Aβ42 and an increased level of tau in the CSF whose postmortem biochemical analysis met the neuropathologic criteria of AD.

An inverse relation between PiB deposition and CSF Aβ42 has been reported.[43] However, low levels of CSF Aβ42 can occur in the absence of increased PiB deposition,[44] possibly because PiB may fail to bind to certain human amyloid confirmations, such as diffuse nonfibrillar plaque or concomitant Aβ oligomer formation. Therefore, although preliminary studies based on clinical diagnosis are encouraging, the precise sensitivity and specificity of PiB-PET for AD pathology need to be determined by further postmortem studies.

Patients with familial AD caused by presenilin-1 mutations show an atypical pattern of PiB deposition, with high uptake in the striatum and low cortical uptake.[45] Striatal binding is found in asymptomatic presenilin-1 mutation carriers, suggesting that striatal amyloid deposition may be an early feature of familial AD.

SUMMARY

PiB-PET shows potential for distinguishing AD from frontotemporal dementia[46] and AD from healthy controls, although specificity for the latter requires further examination. Amyloid imaging in healthy controls may detect those at high risk of future AD, identifying them as candidates for early preventive measures if and when they become available. A promising ^{18}F-labeled imaging marker[47] is currently available, which if successful will allow broader application of amyloid imaging in clinical practice and research. The development of in vivo biomarkers for other critical elements of AD pathogenesis such as soluble Aβ and tau would further inform our understanding of the disease and assist in developing and testing disease-modifying therapies for AD.[48]

REFERENCES

1. Hardy J, Selkoe DJ. The amyloid hypothesis of Alzheimer's disease: progress and problems on the road to therapeutics. Science 2002;297(5580):353–6.
2. Mathis CA, Wang Y, Holt DP, et al. Synthesis and evaluation of ^{11}C-labeled 6-substituted 2-arylbenzothiazoles as amyloid imaging agents. J Med Chem 2003;46(13):2740–54.
3. Klunk WE, Engler H, Nordberg A, et al. Imaging brain amyloid in Alzheimer's disease with Pittsburgh Compound-B. Ann Neurol 2004;55(3):306–19.
4. Bacskai BJ, Frosch MP, Freeman SH, et al. Molecular imaging with Pittsburgh Compound B confirmed at autopsy: a case report. Arch Neurol 2007;64(3):431–4.
5. Ikonomovic MD, Klunk WE, Abrahamson EE, et al. Post-mortem correlates of in vivo PiB-PET amyloid imaging in a typical case of Alzheimer's disease. Brain 2008;131(Pt 6):1630–45.
6. Ng S, Villemagne VL, Berlangieri S, et al. Visual assessment versus quantitative assessment of ^{11}C-PIB PET and ^{18}F-FDG PET for detection of Alzheimer's disease. J Nucl Med 2007;48(4):547–52.
7. Fodero-Tavoletti MT, Rowe CC, McLean CA, et al. Characterization of PiB binding to white matter in Alzheimer disease and other dementias. J Nucl Med 2009;50(2):198–204.
8. Logan J. Graphical analysis of PET data applied to reversible and irreversible tracers. Nucl Med Biol 2000;27(7):661–70.
9. Mintun MA, Larossa GN, Sheline YI, et al. [11]C]PIB in a nondemented population: potential antecedent marker of Alzheimer disease. Neurology 2006;67(3):446–52.
10. Koivunen J, Verkkoniemi A, Aalto S, et al. PET amyloid ligand [11C]PIB uptake shows predominantly striatal increase in variant Alzheimer's disease. Brain 2008;131(Pt 7):1845–53.
11. Lopresti BJ, Klunk WE, Mathis CA, et al. Simplified quantification of Pittsburgh Compound B amyloid imaging PET studies: a comparative analysis. J Nucl Med 2005;46(12):1959–72.
12. McNamee RL, Yee SH, Price JC, et al. Consideration of optimal time window for Pittsburgh compound B PET summed uptake measurements. J Nucl Med 2009;50(3):348–55.
13. Mikhno A, Devanand D, Pelton G, et al. Voxel-based analysis of ^{11}C-PIB scans for diagnosing Alzheimer's disease. J Nucl Med 2008;49(8):1262–9.
14. Villemagne VL, Pike KE, Chételat G, et al. Longitudinal assessment of Aβ and cognition in aging and Alzheimer disease. Ann Neurol 2011;69(1):181–92.
15. Bennett DA, Schneider JA, Arvanitakis Z, et al. Neuropathology of older persons without cognitive impairment from two community-based studies. Neurology 2006;66(12):1837–44.
16. Hulette CM, Welsh-Bohmer KA, Murray MG, et al. Neuropathological and neuropsychological changes in "normal" aging: evidence for preclinical Alzheimer disease in cognitively normal individuals. J Neuropathol Exp Neurol 1998;57(12):1168–74.
17. Pike KE, Savage G, Villemagne VL, et al. Beta-amyloid imaging and memory in non-demented individuals: evidence for preclinical Alzheimer's disease. Brain 2007;130(Pt 11):2837–44.
18. Jack CR Jr, Lowe VJ, Senjem ML, et al. 11C PiB and structural MRI provide complementary information in imaging of Alzheimer's disease and amnestic mild cognitive impairment. Brain 2008;131(Pt 3):665–80.
19. Aizenstein HJ, Nebes RD, Saxton JA, et al. Frequent amyloid deposition without significant cognitive impairment among the elderly. Arch Neurol 2008;65(11):1509–17.
20. Mormino EC, Kluth JT, Madison CM, et al. Episodic memory loss is related to hippocampal-mediated beta-amyloid deposition in elderly subjects. Brain 2009;132(Pt 5):1310–23.
21. Braak H, Braak E. Frequency of stages of Alzheimer-related lesions in different age categories. Neurobiol Aging 1997;18(4):351–7.
22. Rowe CC, Ellis KA, Rimajova M, et al. Amyloid imaging results from the Australian Imaging, Biomarkers and Lifestyle (AIBL) study of aging. Neurobiol Aging 2010;31(8):1275–83.
23. Mosconi L, Rinne JO, Tsui WH, et al. Increased fibrillar amyloid-{beta} burden in normal individuals with a family history of late-onset Alzheimer's. Proc Natl Acad Sci U S A 2010;107(13):5949–54.
24. Reiman EM, Chen K, Liu X, et al. Fibrillar amyloid-beta burden in cognitively normal people at 3 levels of genetic risk for Alzheimer's disease. Proc Natl Acad Sci U S A 2009;106(16):6820–5.
25. Langbaum JB, Chen K, Launer LJ, et al. Blood pressure is associated with higher brain amyloid burden and lower glucose metabolism in healthy late middle-age persons. Neurobiol Aging 2011. [Epub ahead of print].
26. Li NC, Lee A, Whitmer RA, et al. Use of angiotensin receptor blockers and risk of dementia in a predominantly male population: prospective cohort analysis. BMJ 2010;340:b5465.
27. Rowe CC, Ng S, Ackermann U, et al. Imaging beta-amyloid burden in aging and dementia. Neurology 2007;68(20):1718–25.
28. Becker JA, Hedden T, Carmasin J, et al. Amyloid-β associated cortical thinning in clinically normal elderly. Ann Neurol 2011;69(6):1032–42.

29. Oh H, Mormino EC, Madison C, et al. β-Amyloid affects frontal and posterior brain networks in normal aging. Neuroimage 2011;54(3):1887–95.

30. Mormino EC, Smiljic A, Hayenga AO, et al. Relationships between beta-amyloid and functional connectivity in different components of the default mode network in aging. Cereb Cortex 2011;21(10):2399–407.

31. Driscoll I, Zhou Y, An Y, et al. Lack of association between ^{11}C-PiB and longitudinal brain atrophy in non-demented older individuals. Neurobiol Aging 2011;32(12):2123–30.

32. Jack CR Jr, Lowe VJ, Weigand SD, et al. Serial PIB and MRI in normal, mild cognitive impairment and Alzheimer's disease: implications for sequence of pathological events in Alzheimer's disease. Brain 2009;132(Pt 5):1355–65.

33. Sojkova J, Zhou Y, An Y, et al. Longitudinal patterns of β-amyloid deposition in nondemented older adults. Arch Neurol 2011;68(5):644–9.

34. Morris JC, Roe CM, Grant EA, et al. Pittsburgh compound B imaging and prediction of progression from cognitive normality to symptomatic Alzheimer disease. Arch Neurol 2009;66(12):1469–75.

35. St George-Hyslop PH, Morris JC. Will anti-amyloid therapies work for Alzheimer's disease? Lancet 2008;372(9634):180–2.

36. Kemppainen NM, Aalto S, Wilson IA, et al. PET amyloid ligand [11C]PIB uptake is increased in mild cognitive impairment. Neurology 2007;68(19):1603–6.

37. Forsberg A, Engler H, Almkvist O, et al. PET imaging of amyloid deposition in patients with mild cognitive impairment. Neurobiol Aging 2008;29(10):1456–65.

38. Wolk DA, Price JC, Saxton JA, et al. Amyloid imaging in mild cognitive impairment subtypes. Ann Neurol 2009;65(5):557–68.

39. Edison P, Archer HA, Hinz R, et al. Amyloid, hypometabolism, and cognition in Alzheimer disease: an [11C]PIB and [18F]FDG PET study. Neurology 2007;68(7):501–8.

40. Berg L, McKeel DW Jr, Miller JP, et al. Clinicopathologic studies in cognitively healthy aging and Alzheimer's disease: relation of histologic markers to dementia severity, age, sex, and apolipoprotein E genotype. Arch Neurol 1998;55(3):326–35.

41. Leinonen V, Alafuzoff I, Aalto S, et al. Assessment of beta-amyloid in a frontal cortical brain biopsy specimen and by positron emission tomography with carbon 11-labeled Pittsburgh Compound B. Arch Neurol 2008;65(10):1304–9.

42. Cairns NJ, Ikonomovic MD, Benzinger T, et al. Absence of Pittsburgh compound B detection of cerebral amyloid beta in a patient with clinical, cognitive, and cerebrospinal fluid markers of Alzheimer disease: a case report. Arch Neurol 2009; 66(12):1557–62.

43. Fagan AM, Mintun MA, Mach RH, et al. Inverse relation between in vivo amyloid imaging load and cerebrospinal fluid Abeta42 in humans. Ann Neurol 2006;59(3):512–9.

44. Fagan AM, Head D, Shah AR, et al. Decreased cerebrospinal fluid Abeta(42) correlates with brain atrophy in cognitively normal elderly. Ann Neurol 2009;65(2):176–83.

45. Klunk WE, Price JC, Mathis CA, et al. Amyloid deposition begins in the striatum of presenilin-1 mutation carriers from two unrelated pedigrees. J Neurosci 2007;27(23):6174–684.

46. Rabinovici GD, Furst AJ, O'Neil JP, et al. ^{11}C-PIB PET imaging in Alzheimer disease and frontotemporal lobar degeneration. Neurology 2007;68(15): 1205–12.

47. Fleisher AS, Chen K, Liu X, et al. Using positron emission tomography and Florbetapir F 18 to image cortical amyloid in patients with mild cognitive impairment or dementia due to Alzheimer disease. Arch Neurol 2011;68(11):1404–11.

48. Rinne JO, Brooks DJ, Rossor MN, et al. ^{11}C-PiB PET assessment of change in fibrillar amyloid-beta load in patients with Alzheimer's disease treated with bapineuzumab: a phase 2, double-blind, placebo-controlled, ascending-dose study. Lancet Neurol 2010;9(4):363–72.

Neuroimaging of Dementia with Lewy Bodies

John-Paul Taylor, MBBS(Hons), PhD, MRCPsych*,
John O'Brien, MA, DM, FRCPsych

KEYWORDS

- Neuroimaging • Dementia with Lewy bodies
- Differential diagnosis

HISTORY

Dementia with Lewy bodies (DLB) is a relative newcomer to the field of late-life dementia, and its late emergence as an independent disease entity can in part be explained by its history. Friedrich Lewy[1] initially noted the presence of spherical neuronal inclusions in autopsy cases of paralysis agitans, which were later coined Lewy bodies (LBs). Later in 1961, a case report by Okazaki and colleagues[2] described two curious cases of elderly men who presented with dementia but who died shortly after with severe extrapyramidal rigidity, and who at autopsy had widespread LBs in the cerebral cortices. Over the next 20 years, further cases of dementia with parkinsonism were reported by Japanese researchers. Nevertheless, LB dementia was considered a rare condition, with the frequent co-occurrence of Alzheimer's pathology (see later discussion) evident in the autopsy cases. Several competing labels were used, including diffuse LB disease,[3] dementia associated with cortical LBs,[4] the LB variant of Alzheimer's disease (AD),[5] senile dementia of LB type,[6] and LB dementia.[7]

Real interest in DLB, however, emerged in the late 1980s with advances in neuropathologic techniques including ubiquitin staining, which made the visualization of LBs easier. Seminal work done in a series of careful autopsy studies identified that LBs were actually a common feature of late-life dementia, affecting between 15% and 20% of elderly demented cases,[5,6] and thus establishing DLB as the second most common form of degenerative dementia in old age. More recently, specific α-synuclein immunohistochemical staining has shown α-synuclein to be the core element of LBs, therefore placing DLB at the heart of the pathologic family of α-synucleinopathies that includes diseases such as Parkinson disease (PD), the associated Parkinson disease dementia (PDD), multisystem atrophy, pure autonomic failure, and rapid eye movement (REM) sleep behavior disorder. Further advances have shown that small aggregates of α-synuclein, not necessarily associated with LBs, are widespread in the brains of people with DLB, and it has been speculated that these small deposits may directly impair synaptic function, upset neuronal homeostatic energy processing, and lead ultimately to neuronal cell death.[8,9] Nevertheless, linking how the pathologic changes lead to cognitive dysfunction and the other deleterious symptoms in DLB remains unclear.

CLINICAL CHARACTERIZATION

Concordant with advances in neuropathology, research into DLB has led to the clearer clinical characterization of DLB, with the development of operationalized consensus criteria initially published in 1996[10] and revised in 2005 (**Box 1**).[11]

Disclosures: John O'Brien has acted as a consultant to GE Healthcare and Bayer Healthcare. John-Paul Taylor has nothing to disclose.
Institute for Ageing and Health, Wolfson Research Centre, Campus for Aging and Vitality, Newcastle University, Newcastle Upon Tyne, NE4 5PL, UK
* Corresponding author.
E-mail address: john-paul.taylor@ncl.ac.uk

Neuroimag Clin N Am 22 (2012) 67–81
doi:10.1016/j.nic.2011.11.001
1052-5149/12/$ – see front matter © 2012 Elsevier Inc. All rights reserved.

Box 1
Consensus criteria for the clinical diagnosis of probable and possible DLB

1. Central feature (essential for a diagnosis of possible or probable DLB)

   Dementia defined as a progressive cognitive decline of sufficient magnitude to interfere with normal social or occupational function. Prominent or persistent memory impairment may not necessarily occur in the early stages but is usually evident with progression. Deficits on tests of attention, executive function, and visuospatial ability may be especially prominent.

2. Core features (2 core features are sufficient for a diagnosis of probable DLB, 1 for possible DLB)

   a. Fluctuating cognition with pronounced variations in attention and alertness

   b. Recurrent visual hallucinations that are typically well formed and detailed

   c. Spontaneous features of parkinsonism

3. Suggestive features (if one or more of these is present in the presence of one or more core features, a diagnosis of probable DLB can be made)

   In the absence of any core features, one or more suggestive features is sufficient for the diagnosis of possible DLB. Probable DLB should not be diagnosed on the basis of suggestive features alone.

   a. REM sleep behavior disorder

   b. Severe neuroleptic sensitivity

   c. Low dopamine transporter uptake in basal ganglia demonstrated by single-photon emission computed tomography (SPECT) or positron emission tomography (PET) imaging

4. Supportive features (commonly present but not proved to have diagnostic specificity)

   a. Repeated falls and syncope

   b. Transient, unexplained loss of consciousness

   c. Severe autonomic dysfunction, eg, orthostatic hypotension, urinary incontinence

   d. Hallucinations in other modalities

   e. Systematized delusions

   f. Depression

   g. Relative preservation of medial temporal lobe structures on structural imaging

   h. Generalized low uptake on SPECT/PET perfusion scan with reduced occipital activity

   i. Abnormal (low uptake) MIBG myocardial scintigraphy

   j. Prominent slow-wave activity on electroencephalogram with temporal lobe sharp waves

5. A diagnosis of DLB is less likely

   a. In the presence of cerebrovascular disease evident as focal neurologic signs or on brain imaging

   b. In the presence of any other physical illness or brain disorder sufficient to account in part or in total for the clinical picture

   c. If parkinsonism only appears for the first time at a stage of severe dementia

6. Temporal sequence of symptoms

   a. DLB should be diagnosed when dementia occurs before or concurrently with parkinsonism (if present). In research studies, when a distinction needs to be made between DLB and PDD, the 1-year rule between the onset of dementia and parkinsonism should be applied.

Adapted from McKeith IG, Dickson DW, Lowe J, et al. Diagnosis and management of dementia with LBs. Third report of the DLB consortium. Neurology 2005;65:1863–72; with permission.

The criteria clinically define 3 core symptoms for DLB: prominent (vivid) and recurrent visual hallucinations, spontaneous extrapyramidal symptoms, and fluctuating cognitive impairment. Other important clinical features are REM sleep behavior disorder and neuroleptic (antipsychotic) sensitivity. The presence of at least one core symptom plus one of the other supportive features is sufficient to make a diagnosis of probable DLB in the absence of obvious other causes such as cerebrovascular disease. Of note is the significance of neuroimaging in the revised criteria (discussed more in relevant sections in this article). Deficits in striatal dopamine transporter function are strongly suggestive of a diagnosis of DLB; that is, the presence of this plus only one of the core symptoms would be sufficient to make a diagnosis of probable DLB. Supportive neuroimaging features in making a diagnosis of DLB include relative preservation of medial temporal lobe structures on neuroimaging, generalized reductions in perfusion/metabolic imaging with reduced occipital activity, and abnormal cardiac imaging with iodine 123 meta-iodobenzylguanidine ([123I]MIBG).

DIAGNOSIS OF DEMENTIA WITH LBS VERSUS PD WITH DEMENTIA

An area that has been subject to controversy is the separation of DLB from PDD. Consensus criteria for DLB[11] and PDD[12] recommend that for a diagnosis of PDD the extrapyramidal motor features need to be present for at least 12 months or more before the onset of the dementia, but if the dementia precedes the motor symptoms or has occurred within 12 months of the motor features, the diagnosis should be DLB. While subtleties exist between DLB and PDD, both conditions share cognitive, neuropsychiatric, neurochemical, pathologic, and imaging similarities, and this has led to the argument that both PDD and DLB should be considered the same disorder, or at the least two different points on an LB disease spectrum.[13] The arbitrary one-year rule continues to allow distinction for research purposes and understanding the interrelationship between the two disease entities, but clinically, particularly where there is uncertainty concerning the onset of the motor symptoms relative to the cognitive symptoms, unitary approaches should be considered, and the catch-all term of LB dementias that includes both DLB and PDD can be useful in this regard.

DIAGNOSIS OF DLB VERSUS AD

Recognition of DLB is important diagnostically because of the potentially dangerous adverse reaction to neuroleptics, the misuse of antiparkinsonian drugs, and the positive response to cholinesterase inhibitors.[14] It has also been recognized that levels of neuropsychiatric symptomatology, functional disability, impaired quality of life, increased hospitalization, and annual care costs in DLB are significantly greater than those associated with AD,[11,15,16] and thus early and accurate diagnosis is likely to be an essential component of effective treatment and management.

However, despite the development of clinical criteria, it is still apparent that DLB is underdiagnosed. Whereas 15% to 20% of dementia cases demonstrate neuropathologic features of DLB, epidemiologic surveys have tended to show rates of DLB to be much lower, at between 1% and 5%.[17] This discrepancy has in part been driven by the lack of awareness of DLB as an independent clinical entity, difficulties in making the diagnosis clinically, and the interaction between coexistent AD and LB pathologies. Neuropathologically, up to 90% of DLB cases have high senile plaque counts, a level comparable with those found in pure AD, although only a minority of DLB cases show typical AD-associated neocortical neurofibrillary tangles, which are now thought to be integral to the pathophysiology of AD. Amyloid-β in the neocortex has also been associated with more extensive α-synuclein lesions, and thus it has been speculated that amyloid-β may have a role in the genesis of α-synuclein deposition in DLB.[18]

Recent clinicopathologic data have suggested that the expression of a DLB clinical phenotype is related to the severity of LB pathology and inversely related to the severity of Alzheimer-type pathology (Table 1).[19,20] This finding has significant ramifications in making it difficult to diagnose DLB on clinical grounds alone in all cases.

NEUROIMAGING IN DLB

One of the main areas for advancing research and improving the diagnosis of DLB has been the use of imaging, and the following sections explore the use of several imaging modalities that have been applied in DLB. These have focused mainly on imaging of brain structures and function although, given the increasing recognition that DLB is a multisystem disorder, a discussion is included on the use of cardiac imaging with [123I] MIBG to differentially diagnose DLB.

STRUCTURAL MAGNETIC RESONANCE IMAGING

Volumetric changes in dementia, whether global or region specific, can be elucidated using structural magnetic resonance (MR). Although the largest body of literature exists for Alzheimer's dementia, volumetric studies in DLB have helped in defining some of the neurobiological underpinnings of the disease, as well as making important contributions to the differential diagnosis of the condition and providing insights into its longitudinal progression. Analysis of structural data has included several methods ranging from simple visual inspection,

Table 1
Relationship of DLB clinical phenotype to the severity of LB and Alzheimer-type pathologies

| | | Alzheimer-Type Pathology | | |
		NIA-Reagan Low	NIA-Reagan Intermediate	NIA-Reagan High
		(Braak Stage 0–II)	(Braak Stage III–IV)	(Braak Stage V–VI)
LB type pathology	Brainstem predominant	Low	Low	Low
	Limbic (transitional)	High	Intermediate	Low
	Diffuse neocortical	High	High	Intermediate

The likelihood (high, intermediate, or low) that the observed neuropathology explains the typical DLB clinical syndrome (fluctuating cognitive impairment, recurrent visual hallucinations, and parkinsonism) is directly related to the severity of LB-related pathology, and inversely related to the severity of concurrent AD-type pathology.

Abbreviation: NIA-Reagan, National Institute on Aging–Reagan Institute criteria for the neuropathological diagnosis of Alzheimer's disease.

Adapted from McKeith IG, Dickson DW, Lowe J, et al. Diagnosis and management of dementia with Lewy bodies. Third report of the DLB consortium. Neurology 2005;65:1863–72; with permission.

through to region of interest (ROI) analysis and voxel-based morphometry (VBM). ROI and visual rating methods have been very much human led with operator-defined structures of interest, whereas VBM analysis has no a priori biases and makes statistical comparisons on a point-by-point basis (voxel level) across data sets.

Atrophic Changes in DLB

One of the main findings in AD is that of widespread global atrophy. In DLB the findings are less consistent; several studies have reported increased atrophy in DLB (**Fig. 1**) in insular, frontal, inferior parietal, temporal, and occipital cortices compared with similarly aged controls, with relative sparing of the sensorimotor cortex.[21–24] A large study by Whitwell and colleagues[25] found very little cortical atrophy in patients with DLB aside from some subtle cortical loss in frontal and parietal lobes as well as volumetric reductions in hypothalamus, basal forebrain, and midbrain regions. The latter findings have also been reported in DLB by other groups,[26,27] and may explain the marked cholinergic deficits apparent in DLB given that the nucleus basalis of Meynert is contained in the substantia innominata. However, in the studies by Whitwell and colleagues[25] and Hanyu and colleagues,[26] midbrain atrophy was also noted in AD patients, so these changes may not be specific to DLB.

Putamen atrophy has been reported in DLB in comparison with AD by Cousins and colleagues,[28] although no significant structural differences have been found in the caudate nucleus of DLB patients[28,29] in contrast to PDD,[30] where atrophy of the right caudate tail was found in one structural

VBM study.[22] Overall, striatal structural atrophic changes may reflect increased α-synuclein pathology but they probably are less indicative of functional dopaminergic loss in DLB, probably for 2 main reasons. First, Cousins and colleagues[28] did not find a link between striatal atrophy and the severity of motor symptoms, and second, the magnitude of atrophy (5%–10%) is much less marked than the large (50%) reductions that occur in DLB in the uptake of radioligands, which bind to the striatal dopamine transporter (see later discussion).

Overall, therefore, global and subcortical atrophic changes have not proved to be particularly useful in the differential diagnosis of DLB. Perhaps the most consistent finding has been the lack of medial temporal lobe atrophy in DLB compared with AD on both visual inspection (**Fig. 2**) and volumetric analysis,[21,31–33] although the presence of medial temporal atrophy does not rule out a diagnosis of DLB.[34] Instead medial temporal lobe atrophy, if present, tends to rule in AD rather than other dementias; this is supported by an autopsy study of 46 patients with dementia (AD, DLB, and vascular) by Burton and colleagues,[35] who noted that antemortem MR of the medial temporal lobe was robustly associated with Alzheimer tangle pathology rather than plaque or LB pathology within the temporal lobe.

Nevertheless, more recent reports using high-resolution structural MR imaging have suggested that subtleties exist between AD and DLB with regard to hippocampal subfield atrophy.[36] Sabattoli and colleagues[36] noted differential atrophy of more anterior regions in DLB compared with AD, consistent with CA2 and CA3 atrophy, and Firbank and colleagues[37] reported reduced subiculum

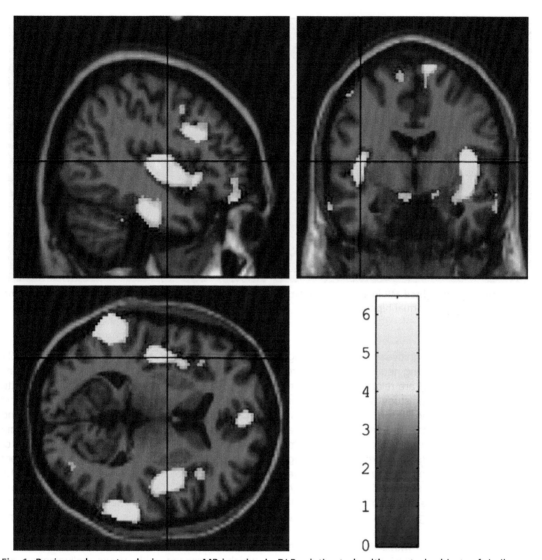

Fig. 1. Regions where atrophy is seen on MR imaging in DLB relative to healthy control subjects of similar age.

thickness, selective CA1 neuronal loss, and loss of distinction in a hypointense line that is visible between CA1 and CA3/4 in AD subjects in comparison with controls. This evidence is preliminary, but if replicated in larger samples high-resolution hippocampal imaging may become an additional tool in making a differential diagnosis between AD and DLB.

Progression of Atrophy in DLB

Several longitudinal studies using serial MR have suggested annual rates of atrophy that are comparable in patients with DLB and AD (approximately 1.5%–2% per year vs 0.5% in controls).[25,38] Nevertheless, the presence of concomitant AD pathology may influence the trajectory of atrophic progression. In the study by Whitwell and

colleagues,[25] patients with pure AD, pure DLB, and mixed AD/DLB pathology were examined; patients with pure DLB had atrophy and ventricular expansion rates comparable with those of aged controls (0.4% and 4.8% per year, respectively) and were lower than subjects with AD (atrophy 1.1% per year with a ventricular expansion rate of 8.3% per year), whereas the mixed AD/DLB group had atrophy levels comparable with those of the AD group (1.3% per year, ventricular expansion 7.2% per year).

Atrophy and Association with Underlying Neuropathology and Clinical Symptoms

Structural MR imaging has also been used in DLB to help understand the relationship between the underlying neuropathology and associated

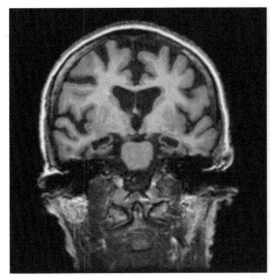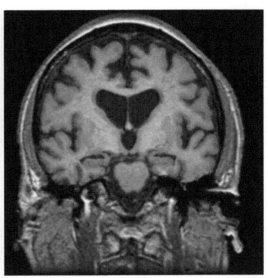

Fig. 2. Coronal T1-weighted MR imaging. (*Left*) Patient with AD showing marked hippocampal atrophy. (*Right*) Patient with DLB with normal hippocampi.

neuropsychiatric and cognitive symptoms, although specific studies examining neuropathologic correlates of atrophy in DLB are relatively sparse. One major neuropathologic study with antemortem structural MR data by Burton and colleagues[39] noted that a significant inverse correlation was observed between normalized amygdala volume and percent area of LBs in the amygdala, although there were no other significant correlations between regional volume and measures of neuropathology.

Cognitive symptoms in DLB may correlate with regional atrophic changes; for example, a comparative VBM study by Sanchez-Castaneda and colleagues[24] of patients with DLB and PDD noted that patients with DLB had greater gray matter loss in frontal areas compared with patients with PDD, and that in patients with DLB prefrontal and anterior cingulate volume correlated with performance scores on a continuous performance test, a measure of sustained attention, whereas right hippocampal and amygdala volume was associated with visual memory function. Hippocampal atrophy (specifically CA1 volume reduction) in DLB was also found to be associated with poor memory function. These hippocampal data suggest that concomitant AD pathology may have a role in DLB in mediating memory dysfunction.

Given the marked visuoperceptual deficits and visual hallucinations that occur in DLB, others have sought to find regional atrophic changes, such as in the occipital lobe, that may relate to these clinical features. Occipital hypometabolism and hypoperfusion in DLB (see later discussion)

have been observed using PET and SPECT imaging[40–42] in DLB, but most volumetric studies using ROI analysis[43] and VBM[21,22] have failed to find any significant occipital structural changes in DLB, although one study using VBM did find more atrophy in the left occipital gyrus in patients with DLB than in controls.[23] Overall, the lack of major occipital atrophy is probably consistent with the lack of significant LB pathology in the occipital pole.[44] Other areas relating to higher visual processing and executive function may be more relevant for visual hallucinations; one recent report noted decreased volume in associative visual areas and the inferior frontal lobe, which correlated with visual hallucinations in DLB.[45]

White Matter Hyperintensities

On T2-weighted and fluid-attenuated inversion recovery (FLAIR) images, white matter lesions (WML) or hyperintensities have been observed in patients with neurodegenerative disease and in healthy older people; pathologically these lesions relate to loss of myelin, axonal damage, and gliosis. Their presence often concords with small vessel disease, and it is presumed that they are a radiologic marker for localized vascular damage. However, the location of these lesions may be relevant; periventricular hyperintensities as opposed to deep white matter lesions correlate with increasing ventricular dilatation in patients with DLB and AD suggesting that, in these cases, the periventricular lesions relate more to atrophy than to vascular ischemia.[46] Nevertheless, findings with regard to WML severity and their occurrence in DLB relative to controls and other neurodegenerative disorders have been inconsistent, and may relate to the analysis method used. Studies using visual rating scales have suggested that WMLs are more extensive in patients with DLB than in control subjects, although levels are similar to that of AD.[46,47] However, another study that used automated quantification methods[48] found no significant difference between the amount of WML in patients with DLB compared with controls and patients with PDD, although both groups had lesser amounts compared with patients with AD. These findings and the current lack of effects of WML on cognitive function in DLB mean that the role and importance of WML in the etiopathology of DLB remains to be resolved.

DIFFUSION MR

Diffusion MR is a methodology that measures the overall direction and magnitude of diffusivity of water molecules in the brain. The underlying premise is that disruption to cellular structures as a consequence of neurodegeneration leads to alterations in water diffusion. Several methods have been devised to measure this phenomenon, including mean diffusivity (MD), which is a measure of the average motion of water molecules independent of any tissue directionality and which depends on cellular structure, and fractional anisotropy (FA), which reflects the tendency of water to move in the same direction within axons and fiber tracts; reductions in the latter measure disruption to axonal integrity. Beyond this, diffusion MR has allowed the characterization of white matter connectivity in the brain (tractography) by examining the principal direction of the diffusion tensor.

Several diffusion MR abnormalities have been reported in DLB, although the findings are not consistent. For example, Bozzali and colleagues[49] found widespread cortical white matter changes with increased MD and decreased FA in callosal and pericallosal areas of 15 DLB patients compared with 10 controls, with further changes in white matter noted in frontal, parietal, and occipital areas, although temporal areas were relatively spared. Subcortical changes in the caudate nucleus and the putamen were also observed. By contrast, the study by Firbank and colleagues[50] noted that although specific FA reductions were observed in precuneus areas on an ROI analysis, the diffuse and widespread changes observed by Bozzali and colleagues were not found. Posterior

changes have also been observed in the related condition of PDD by Matsui and colleagues,[51] who found a reduction in FA in the posterior cingulate (ROI) in PDD subjects compared with PD and control subjects. Firbank and colleagues[52] found a small cluster in the white matter underlying the postcentral gyrus where FA was lower in a DLB group relative to a control group. In subjects with DLB (and also a combined dementia cohort), FA changes were correlated with the motor subscale score of the unified Parkinson disease rating scale (UPDRS). More recent, larger studies[53,54] have found increased MD in the amygdala as well as decreased FA in fiber tracts connected to the occipital pole (eg, inferior longitudinal fasciculus and inferior occipitofrontal fasciculus) in DLB patients in comparison with aged controls, with evidence to suggest that diffusivity deficits in visual-related white matter and amygdala are related to the presence of visual hallucinations and severity of parkinsonism, respectively; nevertheless, the causal explanation of why changes in amygdala diffusivity lead to parkinsonism is not clear. In these studies direct comparison of DLB with AD did not demonstrate any significant differences in diffusion parameters, although diffusion MR may enhance diagnostic discrimination between the disease groups when considered with gray matter density in the amygdala for DLB and hippocampal areas for AD.

In summary, there are some white matter changes evident in DLB on diffusion MR, although these await further characterization, and certainly there are currently insufficient data to determine whether diffusion MR is a viable method to distinguish DLB from other dementias. Nevertheless, the changes seen in diffusion MR in DLB may provide evidence of specific disruptions in white connectivity between associative and motor areas that relate to clinical symptoms of perceptual disturbance and motor dysfunction.

MR SPECTROSCOPY

Neuronal and glial function can be indirectly assessed by measuring the levels of key biomolecules such as N-acetyl aspartate (NAA), glutamine, myo-inositol, and choline with proton MR spectroscopy referenced against creatinine (CR), a marker of general metabolism.

Several studies have used MR spectroscopy in DLB, although results are varied, likely as a result of small sample size and very large voxels of interest (typically $1–8$ cm^3). A general consensus of findings (although not all) suggests a relative preservation of NAA/CR ratios in patients with DLB compared with patients with AD (see Watson and colleagues[55] for discussion). However, the neurobiological basis of these findings still remains to be clarified.

FUNCTIONAL IMAGING OF BRAIN ACTIVITY IN DLB

Examination of blood-flow–related activity changes by using techniques such as PET with $H_2{}^{15}O$ or functional MR (fMR) imaging have provided major insights regarding both health and disease into the spatiotemporal characteristics of dynamic brain processing, including the basis of cognitive function (and dysfunction).

In PD without dementia, several studies have examined executive and working memory function with PET,[56–58] and have focused on understanding the neurobiological basis of visual hallucinations and associated perturbations in cortical visual function.[59–62] However, in DLB there is only one published functional fMR imaging study to date,[63] which found reduced activity in response to moving stimuli compared with patients with AD and aged control subjects. A large barrier, and probably the reason why there are so few data currently available on functional imaging of brain activity in DLB (and a factor for functional imaging studies in other dementias), is the difficulties encountered with getting subjects to engage with the task; it becomes difficult to determine whether activation differences between subjects and controls are disease specific or are more related to hemodynamic response variability arising as a result of degree of engagement/nonengagement in the task by the patient. Functional tasks either need to be essentially passive with minimal cognitive engagement (but thus severely limiting the range of paradigms that could be applied) or need to be adaptive to a subject's performance level to overcome this issue.[64]

Alternatively, functional brain activity has been examined during rest; in normal subjects, diffuse cortical regions show an interrelated increase in activity during rest, with a decrease in activity of these regions or deactivation during a cognitive task. Of these so-called resting-state networks, one of the most commonly described is that of the default mode network (DMN), which includes medial prefrontal cortex, posterior cingulate, medial temporal, and precuneus. In DLB, Sauer and colleagues[63] reported that task-related deactivation of the DMN was decreased in DLB during color and motion tasks, although these deficits were no greater than those observed in patients with AD. Functional resting-state connectivity, that is, the functional correlation in blood oxygen level dependent (BOLD) activity between resting-

state regions has also been examined; a study in a small sample of subjects with DLB using a precuneus seed region found increased resting-state connectivity between this area and the inferior parietal cortex as well as putamen, with decreased connectivity with medial prefrontal, frontoparietal operculum, and visual cortices.[65] There were differences in BOLD functional connectivity in patients with AD, thus it is possible that this methodology may have some promise in the differential diagnosis of DLB. However, the pathophysiological significance of resting-state changes in DLB is still poorly understood and more studies are needed.

PERFUSION/METABOLISM IMAGING

Cerebral glucose metabolism can be indirectly inferred using [^{18}F]fluorodeoxyglucose (FDG)-PET, and brain perfusion can be estimated with SPECT using radiotracers such as [^{99m}Tc]hexamethylpropylene amine oxime (HMPAO), N-isopropyl-p-[^{123}I] iodoamphetamine (IMP), and [^{99m}Tc]ethylcysteinate dimer (ECD). More recently, cerebral perfusion in DLB has been examined using the technique of arterial spin labeling MR (ASL-MR).[66]

Clinically, perhaps the most widely used modality is that of SPECT-HMPAO, with studies focusing on using this method to distinguish between DLB and AD based on the degree of occipital hypoperfusion. However, sensitivity rates across studies have been variable depending on the study (eg, Lobotesis and colleagues,[41] 65%; Shimizu and colleagues,[67] 85%), and occipital hypoperfusion indeed may not be the norm; a recent challenging article by Kemp and colleagues,[68] who used [^{123}I]2β-carbomethoxy-3β-(4-iodophenyl)-N-(3-fluoropropyl)nortropane (FP-CIT) imaging (see later discussion) as a diagnostic gold standard, noted that only 28% of patients with DLB demonstrated occipital hypoperfusion, with a similar proportion (31%) of patients with non-DLB dementia demonstrating occipital hypoperfusion.

Clinically, SPECT perfusion is probably inferior to MIBG[69,70] and FP-CIT imaging[71] in DLB diagnosis in terms of sensitivity and specificity. One of the drivers undermining the use of SPECT perfusion imaging may be the low spatial resolution of this modality; this is supported by a comparative study between FDG-PET and SPECT-IMP, which found PET to be more sensitive than SPECT-IMP to the occipital hypometabolism.[72] Nevertheless, even PET studies are not entirely consistent[73]; although occipital hypometabolism is mostly reported, greater parietal than occipital hypometabolism has also been observed in DLB.[72]

Whether cognition relates to perfusion/metabolism changes in DLB is not clear. Although Colloby and colleagues[74] successfully demonstrated a positive correlation between Mini-Mental State Examination (MMSE) score and temporoparietal blood flow in AD, they failed to find a similar relationship in DLB, which they speculated to be related to potential floor effects in DLB due to marked parietal hypoperfusion or lack of sensitivity of the MMSE as a cognitive measure in DLB. However, psychotic symptom clusters in DLB do seem to relate to spatially distinct perfusion deficits. A factor analysis paradigm of Nagahama and colleagues[75] found that delusional phenomenology in DLB concords with frontal hypoperfusion, visual hallucinations with parietal and occipital association cortices perfusion deficits, and delusional misidentifications to hypoperfusion of the limbic-paralimbic structures. Similarly, over a 1-year period, O'Brien and colleagues[76] reported that, in patients with DLB, increased fluctuations in consciousness were linked to increased thalamic and decreased inferior occipital perfusion, whereas increased midline posterior cingulate perfusion was related to reductions in visual hallucinations.

Longitudinal changes in brain perfusion using HMPAO-SPECT have been observed in DLB, with evidence of an increase in striatal perfusion over 1 year that was associated with worsening of parkinsonism, and this change has been speculated to be related to a progressive decline in striatal dopaminergic input. Therapeutic effects have also been measured in DLB using perfusion and metabolic imaging. One report using HMPAO-SPECT[77] with chronic administration of donepezil, a cholinesterase inhibitor, found increased occipital perfusion that was associated with an improvement in visual hallucinations. In another study using ASL-MR imaging,[66] an acute donepezil challenge led to widespread increases in perfusion bilaterally (temporal, parietal, and occipital regions); those subjects who showed the greatest perfusion increase had more marked improvements on a cognitive measure that included attention, working memory, and language function. However, a contrary PET study of patients with DLB who received donepezil for 3 months found that occipital metabolism actually decreased and that this decrease, particularly in the medial and lateral occipital cortices, was related to the degree of improvement in the severity of visual hallucinations in treated subjects. Aside from weaknesses involving sample size and the lack of a control group in this study, explaining this finding versus the contrasting SPECT data is difficult, as there is a lack of knowledge about the way cholinesterase treatments influence the pathophysiology of symptoms such as visual hallucinations, and

precisely how cerebral blood flow relates to brain metabolism in DLB.

In summary, marked perfusion and metabolism deficits have been observed in DLB, particularly posteriorly, and these imaging modalities can be used to distinguish DLB from AD although sensitivity and specificity vary. In addition, understanding how findings of perfusion and metabolism imaging relate to the underlying neurobiology of DLB and its symptoms remains to be understood. Overall, considering only regionally specific reductions in hypoperfusion/metabolism may not necessarily be the best diagnostic method. More relevant may be how these regionally specific reductions arise and co-vary in the context of alterations in the activity of global brain networks. From this perspective application of covariance methodologies may be helpful; certainly in PD they have provided interesting insights into the underlying neurobiology of cognitive dysfunction and symptoms in this condition.[72] The use of covariant ROI network analysis of perfusion data in DLB versus AD may offer an increase in sensitivity and specificity above and beyond diagnostic determination of DLB based purely on occipital reductions in blood flow.[78]

DOPAMINERGIC IMAGING

Dopaminergic function in DLB has been examined using both PET and SPECT imaging.[79,80] The latter has gained clinical ascendency with the dopaminergic presynaptic ligand FP-CIT as the investigative modality of choice in distinguishing DLB from AD, so much so that it is embedded as a strongly supportive diagnostic feature in the revised consensus criteria for DLB.[11] Why this is the case is explained here.

In healthy subjects and in patients with AD, FP-CIT is readily taken up in the caudate and putamen, whereas in DLB uptake is almost absent in the putamen and markedly reduced in the caudate (Fig. 3). Several major studies have demonstrated that the presence of an abnormal FP-CIT scan has very good diagnostic accuracy for DLB/PDD, with a sensitivity/specificity of approximately 80% to 90%.[81–83] As a result, in the United Kingdom, the National Institute for Health and Clinical Excellence has recommended the use of FP-CIT SPECT imaging when the diagnosis of DLB is in doubt, and internationally, the European Federation of Neurological Societies guidelines have also recommended the use of dopaminergic SPECT to differentiate between DLB and AD.

Perhaps even more clinically relevant is the potential promise FP-CIT may have in diagnosing clinically uncertain DLB cases. In a 1-year follow-up

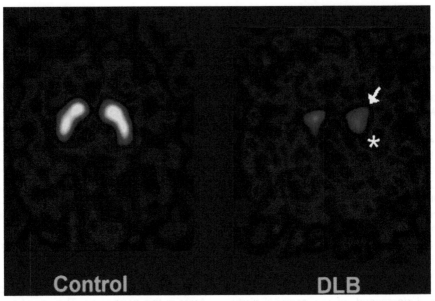

Fig. 3. FP-CIT scan (axial slice through basal ganglia) of a control and a DLB subject, showing reduced dopamine transporter density in the caudate (*arrow*) and putamen (*asterisk*).

study of 44 patients with a baseline diagnosis of possible DLB (ie, only one core symptom or one or more supportive symptoms), O'Brien and colleagues[84] noted that in 26 of these patients (59%) the diagnosis was subsequently revised, with 19 (43%) changed to a diagnosis of probable DLB and 7 (16%) to AD. Among those who at follow-up were diagnosed with probable DLB, 12 had abnormal scans at baseline (sensitivity 63%), and all 7 individuals with a possible diagnosis of DLB at baseline who were subsequently diagnosed as having AD had normal scans (specificity 100%). Thus, an abnormal FP-CIT scan in a person with possible DLB is strongly suggestive of DLB, whereas a normal scan will tend to rule out the diagnosis. In support of this, a study by Walker and colleagues[83] in cases of DLB confirmed post mortem demonstrated that FP-CIT imaging was more accurate than even expert clinical diagnosis in distinguishing DLB from non-LB dementia.

FP-CIT imaging may also provide some clues as to neurobiological changes that occur in DLB. Correlates between striatal FP-CIT uptake and symptoms such as depression, anxiety, apathy, and daytime somnolence have been reported in PD,[85–87] which may reflect the disruption to mesocortical dopaminergic projections from the midbrain to widespread cortical areas. In DLB, Roselli and colleagues[88] noted significant associations between decreased striatal FP-CIT uptake and the severity and frequency of visual hallucinations and caudate uptake was related inversely to delusions, depression, and apathy.

CHOLINERGIC IMAGING

The cholinergic system is intimately involved in cognition, in particular memory, as well as attention and arousal. Unsurprisingly, postmortem studies have shown that profound cholinergic neuronal loss as well as reduced choline acetyltransferase (the presynaptic synthetic enzyme for acetylcholine) activity occurs in DLB. These deficits are even more marked than those seen in AD,[89,90] with widespread cortical and subcortical disturbances of both nicotinic and muscarinic receptors. Treatment of the cholinergic deficit using cholinesterase inhibitors remains the mainstay of treatment for both DLB and AD.

PET imaging using radiolabeled acetylcholine analogues has provided indirect estimation of acetylcholinesterase activity. Differential activity has been observed in patients with DLB in comparison with patients with AD; reductions in activity are seen in the medial occipital cortex of patients with DLB and deficits in the temporal lobe in patients with AD.[91,92]

SPECT imaging has been used to examine muscarinic receptors ([^{123}I]iodo-quinuclidinyl-benzylate or QNB)[93] and nicotinic receptors ([^{125}I]5-iodo-3-[2(S)-2-azetidinylmethoxy]pyridine or 5IA-85380).[94,95] Reductions in uptake in both receptor groups have been observed the frontal and temporal areas in patients with DLB, with increases seen in the occipital pole.

Thus far, the utility of cholinergic radioligands in the differential diagnosis of DLB remains unknown, although they have provided some clues as to the basis of neuropsychiatric symptoms; for example, nicotinic receptor increases in the visual system seem to be higher in patients with DLB who have experienced recent hallucinations,[94] and nicotinic receptor increases in frontal areas also seem to correlate with longitudinal decline in executive function in pooled samples of patients with dementia, inclusive of patients with DLB.[95]

More recently, in vivo visualization of binding of acetylcholinesterase inhibitors in AD has been demonstrated using the PET radioligand [5-^{11}C-methoxy]donepezil[96]; application of this technique in a DLB cohort may provide further elucidation of the cause of cholinergic dysfunction in this population.

CARDIAC IMAGING

Loss of sympathetic innervation to the heart occurs in patients across the LB disease spectrum,[97,98] and this can be measured with [^{123}I] MIBG, an analogue of noradrenaline, with a ratio of heart to mediastinum uptake of this radioligand providing quantification of the degree of sympathetic innervation.

Remarkable accuracies for MIBG in distinguishing DLB from AD have been reported across a range of studies (see Sinha and colleagues[73] for discussion) with sensitivities and specificities of approximately 90%. Furthermore, MIBG uptakes seem to be insensitive to disease duration or severity (see, eg, Refs.[69,99]).

Nevertheless, these studies have been performed mainly on Japanese cohorts, and larger group sizes are needed to confirm the diagnostic accuracy. Other confounders may be reduced uptake in some patients with AD and the effects of comorbid cardiovascular disease.[100] Further research is needed, although MIBG potentially could be a very powerful imaging method in the DLB diagnostic toolbox.

AMYLOID IMAGING

In the AD literature, use of PET tracers that bind to amyloid protein, in particular N-methyl-[^{11}C]2-(4'-methylaminophenyl)-6-hydroxybenzothiazole, also known as Pittsburgh compound B (PIB), has radically changed research approaches to this condition and has provided fundamental insights into disease progression, diagnosis, and neurobiology of AD.

In DLB, autopsy data have often indicated significant comorbid AD pathology although, compared with AD, plaques are more often diffuse than neuritic.[101] This finding has been confirmed in PET studies in DLB, where PIB uptake is increased and comparable with that of AD.[102,103] By contrast, in patients with PDD, uptake is generally similar to controls and patients with PDD alone. From these findings, 2 points emerge: (1) amyloid deposition may have a role in the timing of dementia relative to the motor symptoms of parkinsonism in DLB and PDD; and (2) although amyloid imaging may help discriminate AD from PDD, its clinical utility in differentiating DLB from AD is limited.

Further work is clearly needed, and the greater availability of other amyloid-binding ligands based on ^{18}F, which have longer half-lives and thus can be used at PET centers lacking cyclotrons, may allow for more intensive determination of the use of amyloid-based radioligands as biomarkers in DLB.

SUMMARY

A diversity of imaging methodologies now exists and these have been applied extensively in dementia, particularly AD. By contrast, there are fewer studies on DLB, although methods have yielded fascinating and important insights into the underlying pathophysiology of this condition as well as allowing clinical differentiation of DLB from other dementias, particularly in the case of FP-CIT. The contribution of imaging research to DLB has had significant ramifications in terms of raising the profile of DLB and helping define it as a distinctive and separate disease entity from AD. Further application of established and emerging imaging methods and technologies will undoubtedly make further and significant inroads into the diagnosis and understanding of this condition.

REFERENCES

1. Lewy FH. Paralyis Agitans: I. Pathologische Anatomie. In: Lewandowsky M, editor, Handbuch der Neurologie, vol. 3. Berlin: Julius Springer; 1912. p. 920–33.
2. Okazaki H, Lipton LS, Aronson SM. Diffuse intracytoplasmatic ganglionic inclusions (Lewy type) associated with progressive dementia and quadriparesis in flexion. J Neuropathol Exp Neurol 1961; 20:237–44.
3. Dickson DW, Davies P, Mayeux R, et al. Diffuse Lewy body disease. Neuropathological and biochemical studies of six patients. Acta Neuropathol 1987;75(1):8–15.
4. Byrne EJ, Lowe J, Godwin-Austen RB, et al. Dementia and Parkinson's disease associated with diffuse cortical Lewy bodies. Lancet 1987; 1(8531):501.

5. Hansen L, Salmon D, Galasko D, et al. The Lewy body variant of Alzheimer's disease: a clinical and pathologic entity. Neurology 1990;40(1):1–8.

6. Perry RH, Irving D, Blessed G, et al. Senile dementia of Lewy body type. A clinically and neuropathologically distinct form of Lewy body dementia in the elderly. J Neurol Sci 1990;95(2):119–39.

7. Gibb WR, Esiri MM, Lees AJ. Clinical and pathological features of diffuse cortical Lewy body disease (Lewy body dementia). Brain 1987;110(Pt 5):1131–53.

8. Schulz-Schaeffer W. The synaptic pathology of α-synuclein aggregation in dementia with Lewy bodies, Parkinson's disease and Parkinson's disease dementia. Acta Neuropathol 2010;120(2):131–43.

9. Kramer ML, Schulz-Schaeffer WJ. Presynaptic {alpha}-synuclein aggregates, not Lewy bodies, cause neurodegeneration in dementia with Lewy bodies. J Neurosci 2007;27(6):1405–10.

10. McKeith IG, Galasko D, Kosaka K, et al. Consensus guidelines for the clinical and pathologic diagnosis of dementia with Lewy bodies (DLB): report of the consortium on DLB international workshop. Neurology 1996;47(5):1113–24.

11. McKeith IG, Dickson DW, Lowe J, et al. Diagnosis and management of dementia with Lewy bodies. Third report of the DLB consortium. Neurology 2005;65:1863–72.

12. Emre M, Aarsland D, Brown R, et al. Clinical diagnostic criteria for dementia associated with Parkinson's disease. Mov Disord 2007;22(12):1689–707.

13. Aarsland D, Ballard CG, Halliday G. Are Parkinson's disease with dementia and dementia with Lewy bodies the same entity? J Geriatr Psychiatry Neurol 2004;17(3):137–45.

14. McKeith I, Del Ser T, Spano P, et al. Efficacy of rivastigmine in dementia with Lewy bodies: a randomised, double-blind, placebo-controlled international study. Lancet 2000;356(9247):2031–6.

15. Hanyu H, Sato T, Hirao K, et al. Differences in clinical course between dementia with Lewy bodies and Alzheimer's disease. Eur J Neurol 2009;16(2):212–7.

16. Bostrom F, Jonsson L, Minthon L, et al. Patients with dementia with Lewy bodies have more impaired quality of life than patients with Alzheimer disease. Alzheimer Dis Assoc Disord 2007;21(2):150–4.

17. Zaccai J, McCracken C, Brayne C. A systematic review of prevalence and incidence studies of dementia with Lewy bodies. Age Ageing 2005;34(6):561–6.

18. Pletnikova O, West N, Lee MK, et al. A[beta] deposition is associated with enhanced cortical [alpha]-synuclein lesions in Lewy body diseases. Neurobiol Aging 2005;26(8):1183–92.

19. Kouhei F, Kensuke S, Kazuhito N, et al. Clinicopathological outline of dementia with Lewy bodies applying the revised criteria: the Hisayama study. Brain Pathol 2008;18(3):317–25.

20. McKeith I. Dementia with Lewy bodies and Parkinson's disease with dementia: where two worlds collide. Pract Neurol 2007;7(6):374–82.

21. Burton EJ, Karas G, Paling SM, et al. Patterns of cerebral atrophy in dementia with Lewy bodies using voxel-based morphometry. Neuroimage 2002;17(2):618–30.

22. Burton EJ, McKeith IG, Burn DJ, et al. Cerebral atrophy in Parkinson's disease with and without dementia: a comparison with Alzheimer's disease, dementia with Lewy bodies and controls. Brain 2004;127(Pt 4):791–800.

23. Beyer MK, Larsen JP, Aarsland D. Gray matter atrophy in Parkinson disease with dementia and dementia with Lewy bodies. Neurology 2007;69(8):747–54.

24. Sanchez-Castaneda C, Rene R, Ramirez-Ruiz B, et al. Correlations between gray matter reductions and cognitive deficits in dementia with Lewy Bodies and Parkinson's disease with dementia. Mov Disord 2009;24(12):1740–6.

25. Whitwell JL, Weigand SD, Shiung MM, et al. Focal atrophy in dementia with Lewy bodies on MRI: a distinct pattern from Alzheimer's disease. Brain 2007;130(3):708–19.

26. Hanyu H, Shimizu S, Tanaka Y, et al. MR features of the substantia innominata and therapeutic implications in dementias. Neurobiol Aging 2007;28(4):548–54.

27. Brenneis C, Wenning GK, Egger KE, et al. Basal forebrain atrophy is a distinctive pattern in dementia with Lewy bodies. Neuroreport 2004;15(11):1711–4.

28. Cousins DA, Burton EJ, Burn D, et al. Atrophy of the putamen in dementia with Lewy bodies but not Alzheimer's disease: an MRI study. Neurology 2003;61(9):1191–5.

29. Barber R, McKeith I, Ballard C, et al. Volumetric MRI study of the caudate nucleus in patients with dementia with Lewy bodies, Alzheimer's disease, and vascular dementia. J Neurol Neurosurg Psychiatry 2002;72(3):406–7.

30. Almeida OP, Burton EJ, McKeith I, et al. MRI study of caudate nucleus volume in Parkinson's disease with and without dementia with Lewy bodies and Alzheimer's disease. Dement Geriatr Cogn Disord 2003;16(2):57–63.

31. Barber R, Ballard C, McKeith IG, et al. MRI volumetric study of dementia with Lewy bodies: a comparison with AD and vascular dementia. Neurology 2000;54(6):1304–9.

32. Barber R, McKeith IG, Ballard C, et al. A comparison of medial and lateral temporal lobe atrophy in dementia with Lewy bodies and Alzheimer's disease: magnetic resonance imaging volumetric study. Dement Geriatr Cogn Disord 2001;12(3):198–205.

33. Tam CW, Burton EJ, McKeith IG, et al. Temporal lobe atrophy on MRI in Parkinson disease with dementia: a comparison with Alzheimer disease and dementia with Lewy bodies. Neurology 2005; 64(5):861–5.

34. Barkhof F, Polvikoski TM, van Straaten EC, et al. The significance of medial temporal lobe atrophy: a postmortem MRI study in the very old. Neurology 2007;69(15):1521–7.

35. Burton EJ, Barber R, Mukaetova-Ladinska EB, et al. Medial temporal lobe atrophy on MRI differentiates Alzheimer's disease from dementia with Lewy bodies and vascular cognitive impairment: a prospective study with pathological verification of diagnosis. Brain 2009;132(1):195–203.

36. Sabattoli F, Boccardi M, Galluzzi S, et al. Hippocampal shape differences in dementia with Lewy bodies. Neuroimage 2008;41(3):699–705.

37. Firbank MJ, Blamire AM, Teodorczuk A, et al. High resolution imaging of the medial temporal lobe in Alzheimer's disease and dementia with Lewy bodies. J Alzheimers Dis 2010;21(4):1129–40.

38. O'Brien JT, Paling S, Barber R, et al. Progressive brain atrophy on serial MRI in dementia with Lewy bodies, AD, and vascular dementia. Neurology 2001;56(10):1386–8.

39. Burton EJ, Mukaetova-Ladinska EB, Perry RH, et al. Neuropathological correlates of volumetric MRI in autopsy-confirmed Lewy body dementia. Neurobiol Aging 2011. [Epub ahead of print].

40. Ishii K, Yamaji S, Kitagaki H, et al. Regional cerebral blood flow difference between dementia with Lewy bodies and AD. Neurology 1999;53(2): 413–6.

41. Lobotesis K, Fenwick JD, Phipps A, et al. Occipital hypoperfusion on SPECT in dementia with Lewy bodies but not AD. Neurology 2001;56(5):643–9.

42. Minoshima S, Foster NL, Petrie EC, et al. Neuroimaging in dementia with Lewy bodies: metabolism, neurochemistry, and morphology. J Geriatr Psychiatry Neurol 2002;15(4):200–9.

43. Middelkoop HA, van der Flier WM, Burton EJ, et al. Dementia with Lewy bodies and AD are not associated with occipital lobe atrophy on MRI. Neurology 2001;57(11):2117–20.

44. Gomez-Tortosa E, Newell K, Irizarry MC, et al. Clinical and quantitative pathologic correlates of dementia with Lewy bodies. Neurology 1999; 53(6):1284–91.

45. Sanchez-Castaneda C, Rene R, Ramirez-Ruiz B, et al. Frontal and associative visual areas related to visual hallucinations in dementia with Lewy bodies and Parkinson's disease with dementia. Mov Disord 2010;25(5):615–22.

46. Barber R, Gholkar A, Scheltens P, et al. MRI volumetric correlates of white matter lesions in dementia with Lewy bodies and Alzheimer's disease. Int J Geriatr Psychiatry 2000;15(10):911–6.

47. Barber R, Scheltens P, Gholkar A, et al. White matter lesions on magnetic resonance imaging in dementia with Lewy bodies, Alzheimer's disease, vascular dementia, and normal aging. J Neurol Neurosurg Psychiatry 1999;67(1):66–72.

48. Burton EJ, McKeith IG, Burn DJ, et al. Progression of white matter hyperintensities in Alzheimer disease, dementia with Lewy bodies, and Parkinson disease dementia: a comparison with normal aging. Am J Geriatr Psychiatry 2006;14(10):842–9.

49. Bozzali M, Falini A, Cercignani M, et al. Brain tissue damage in dementia with Lewy bodies: an in vivo diffusion tensor MRI study. Brain 2005;128(Pt 7): 1595–604.

50. Firbank MJ, Blamire AM, Krishnan MS, et al. Diffusion tensor imaging in dementia with Lewy bodies and Alzheimer's disease. Psychiatry Res 2007; 155(2):135–45.

51. Matsui H, Nishinaka K, Oda M, et al. Depression in Parkinson's disease. Diffusion tensor imaging study. J Neurol 2007;254(9):1170–3.

52. Firbank MJ, Blamire AM, Teodorczuk A, et al. Diffusion tensor imaging in Alzheimer's disease and dementia with Lewy bodies. Psychiatry Res 2011; 194(2):176–83.

53. Kiuchi K, Morikawa M, Taoka T, et al. White matter changes in dementia with Lewy bodies and Alzheimer's disease: a tractography-based study. J Psychiatr Res 2011;45(8):1095–100.

54. Kantarci K, Avula R, Senjem ML, et al. Dementia with Lewy bodies and Alzheimer disease: neurodegenerative patterns characterized by DTI. Neurology 2010;74(22):1814–21.

55. Watson R, Blamire AM, O'Brien JT. Magnetic resonance imaging in Lewy body dementias. Dement Geriatr Cogn Disord 2009;28(6):493–506.

56. Owen AM, Doyon J, Dagher A, et al. Abnormal basal ganglia outflow in Parkinson's disease identified with PET. Implications for higher cortical functions. Brain 1998;121(Pt 5):949–65.

57. Thiel A, Hilker R, Kessler J, et al. Activation of basal ganglia loops in idiopathic Parkinson's disease: a PET study. J Neural Transm 2003;110(11): 1289–301.

58. Lewis SJ, Dove A, Robbins TW, et al. Cognitive impairments in early Parkinson's disease are accompanied by reductions in activity in frontostriatal neural circuitry. J Neurosci 2003;23(15):6351–6.

59. Holroyd S, Wooten GF. Preliminary fMRI evidence of visual system dysfunction in Parkinson's disease

patients with visual hallucinations. J Neuropsychiatry Clin Neurosci 2006;18(3):402–4.

60. Meppelink AM, de Jong BM, Renken R, et al. Impaired visual processing preceding image recognition in Parkinson's disease patients with visual hallucinations. Brain 2009;132(11):2980–93.

61. Ramírez-Ruiz B, Martí M-J, Tolosa E, et al. Brain response to complex visual stimuli in Parkinson's patients with hallucinations: a functional magnetic resonance imaging study. Mov Disord 2008; 23(16):2335–43.

62. Stebbins GT, Goetz CG, Carrillo MC, et al. Altered cortical visual processing in PD with hallucinations: an fMRI study. Neurology 2004;63(8): 1409–16.

63. Sauer J, ffytche DH, Ballard C, et al. Differences between Alzheimer's disease and dementia with Lewy bodies: an fMRI study of task-related brain activity. Brain 2006;129(Pt 7):1780–8.

64. Wood JS, Firbank MJ, Mosimann UP, et al. Development of a novel FMRI compatible visual perception prototype battery to test older people with and without dementia. J Geriatr Psychiatry Neurol 2011; 24(2):73–83.

65. Galvin JE, Price JL, Yan Z, et al. Resting bold fMRI differentiates dementia with Lewy bodies vs Alzheimer disease. Neurology 2011;76(21): 1797–803.

66. Fong T, Inouye S, Dai W, et al. Association cortex hypoperfusion in mild dementia with Lewy bodies: a potential indicator of cholinergic dysfunction? Brain Imaging Behav 2010;5(1): 25–35.

67. Shimizu S, Hanyu H, Kanetaka H, et al. Differentiation of dementia with Lewy bodies from Alzheimer's disease using brain SPECT. Dement Geriatr Cogn Disord 2005;20(1):25–30.

68. Kemp PM, Hoffmann SA, Tossici-Bolt L, et al. Limitations of the HMPAO SPECT appearances of occipital lobe perfusion in the differential diagnosis of dementia with Lewy bodies. Nucl Med Commun 2007;28(6):451–6.

69. Hanyu H, Shimizu S, Hirao K, et al. Comparative value of brain perfusion SPECT and [123I]MIBG myocardial scintigraphy in distinguishing between dementia with Lewy bodies and Alzheimer's disease. Eur J Nucl Med Mol Imaging 2006;33(3):248–53.

70. Tateno M, Kobayashi S, Shirasaka T, et al. Comparison of the usefulness of brain perfusion SPECT and MIBG myocardial scintigraphy for the diagnosis of dementia with Lewy bodies. Dement Geriatr Cogn Disord 2008;26(5):453–7.

71. Colloby SJ, Firbank MJ, Pakrasi S, et al. A comparison of 99mTc-exametazime and 123I-FP-CIT SPECT imaging in the differential diagnosis of Alzheimer's disease and dementia with Lewy bodies. Int Psychogeriatr 2008;20(6):1124–40.

72. Ishii K, Hosaka K, Mori T, et al. Comparison of FDG-PET and IMP-SPECT in patients with dementia with Lewy bodies. Ann Nucl Med 2004; 18(5):447–51.

73. Sinha N, Firbank M, O'Brien JT. Biomarkers in dementia with Lewy bodies: a review. Int J Geriatr Psychiatry 2011. [Epub ahead of print].

74. Colloby SJ, Fenwick JD, Williams ED, et al. A comparison of (99m)Tc-HMPAO SPET changes in dementia with Lewy bodies and Alzheimer's disease using statistical parametric mapping. Eur J Nucl Med Mol Imaging 2002;29(5):615–22.

75. Nagahama Y, Okina T, Suzuki N, et al. Neural correlates of psychotic symptoms in dementia with Lewy bodies. Brain 2010;133(Pt 2):557–67.

76. O'Brien JT, Firbank MJ, Mosimann UP, et al. Change in perfusion, hallucinations and fluctuations in consciousness in dementia with Lewy bodies. Psychiatry Res 2005;139(2):79–88.

77. Mori T, Ikeda M, Fukuhara R, et al. Correlation of visual hallucinations with occipital rCBF changes by donepezil in DLB. Neurology 2006;66(6): 935–7.

78. Colloby SJ, Taylor JP, Firbank MJ, et al. Covariance 99mTc-exametazime SPECT patterns in Alzheimer's disease and dementia with Lewy bodies: utility in differential diagnosis. J Geriatr Psychiatry Neurol 2010;23(1):54–62.

79. Hu XS, Okamura N, Arai H, et al. 18F-fluorodopa PET study of striatal dopamine uptake in the diagnosis of dementia with Lewy bodies. Neurology 2000;55(10):1575–7.

80. O'Brien JT, Colloby S, Fenwick J, et al. Dopamine transporter loss visualized with FP-CIT SPECT in the differential diagnosis of dementia with Lewy bodies. Arch Neurol 2004;61(6):919–25.

81. Marshall VL, Patterson J, Hadley DM, et al. Two-year follow-up in 150 consecutive cases with normal dopamine transporter imaging. Nucl Med Commun 2006;27(12):933–7.

82. McKeith I, O'Brien J, Walker Z, et al. Sensitivity and specificity of dopamine transporter imaging with 123I-FP-CIT SPECT in dementia with Lewy bodies: a phase III, multicentre study. Lancet Neurol 2007;6(4):305–13.

83. Walker Z, Jaros E, Walker RW, et al. Dementia with Lewy bodies: a comparison of clinical diagnosis, FP-CIT single photon emission computed tomography imaging and autopsy. J Neurol Neurosurg Psychiatry 2007;78(11):1176–81.

84. O'Brien JT, McKeith IG, Walker Z, et al. Diagnostic accuracy of 123I-FP-CIT SPECT in possible dementia with Lewy bodies. Br J Psychiatry 2009; 194(1):34–9.

85. Murai T, Muller U, Werheid K, et al. In vivo evidence for differential association of striatal dopamine and midbrain serotonin systems with neuropsychiatric

symptoms in Parkinson's disease. J Neuropsychiatry Clin Neurosci 2001;13(2):222–8.

86. Weintraub D, Newberg AB, Cary MS, et al. Striatal dopamine transporter imaging correlates with anxiety and depression symptoms in Parkinson's disease. J Nucl Med 2005;46(2):227–32.

87. Happe S, Baier PC, Helmschmied K, et al. Association of daytime sleepiness with nigrostriatal dopaminergic degeneration in early Parkinson's disease. J Neurol 2007;254(8):1037–43.

88. Roselli F, Pisciotta NM, Perneczky R, et al. Severity of neuropsychiatric symptoms and dopamine transporter levels in dementia with Lewy bodies: a ^{123}I-FP-CIT SPECT study. Mov Disord 2009; 24(14):2097–103.

89. Tiraboschi P, Hansen LA, Alford M, et al. Cholinergic dysfunction in diseases with Lewy bodies. Neurology 2000;54(2):407–11.

90. Tiraboschi P, Hansen LA, Alford M, et al. Early and widespread cholinergic losses differentiate dementia with Lewy bodies from Alzheimer disease. Arch Gen Psychiatry 2002;59(10):946–51.

91. Bohnen NI, Kaufer DI, Ivanco LS, et al. Cortical cholinergic function is more severely affected in parkinsonian dementia than in Alzheimer disease: an in vivo positron emission tomographic study. Arch Neurol 2003;60(12):1745–8.

92. Shimada HM, Hirano SM, Shinotoh HM, et al. Mapping of brain acetylcholinesterase alterations in Lewy body disease by PET. Neurology 2009; 73(4):273–8.

93. Colloby SJ, Pakrasi S, Firbank MJ, et al. In vivo SPECT imaging of muscarinic acetylcholine receptors using (R,R) ^{123}I-QNB in dementia with Lewy bodies and Parkinson's disease dementia. Neuroimage 2006;33(2):423–9.

94. O'Brien JT, Colloby SJ, Pakrasi S, et al. Nicotinic [alpha]4[beta]2 receptor binding in dementia with Lewy bodies using [123]I-5IA-85380 SPECT demonstrates a link between occipital changes and visual hallucinations. Neuroimage 2008; 40(3):1056–63.

95. Colloby SJ, Perry EK, Pakrasi S, et al. Nicotinic [123]I-5IA-85380 single photon emission computed tomography as a predictor of cognitive progression in Alzheimer's disease and dementia with Lewy bodies. Am J Geriatr Psychiatry 2010;18(1):86–90.

96. Okamura N, Funaki Y, Tashiro M, et al. In vivo visualization of donepezil binding in the brain of patients with Alzheimer's disease. Br J Clin Pharmacol 2008;65(4):472–9.

97. Spiegel J, Mollers MO, Jost WH, et al. FP-CIT and MIBG scintigraphy in early Parkinson's disease. Mov Disord 2005;20(5):552–61.

98. Allan LM, Ballard CG, Allen J, et al. Autonomic dysfunction in dementia. J Neurol Neurosurg Psychiatry 2007;78(7):671–7.

99. Yoshita M, Taki J, Yamada M. A clinical role for [(123)I]MIBG myocardial scintigraphy in the distinction between dementia of the Alzheimer's-type and dementia with Lewy bodies. J Neurol Neurosurg Psychiatry 2001;71(5):583–8.

100. Nagayama H, Hamamoto M, Ueda M, et al. Reliability of MIBG myocardial scintigraphy in the diagnosis of Parkinson's disease. J Neurol Neurosurg Psychiatry 2005;76(2):249–51.

101. Ballard C, Ziabreva I, Perry R, et al. Differences in neuropathologic characteristics across the Lewy body dementia spectrum. Neurology 2006;67(11): 1931–4.

102. Gomperts SN, Rentz DM, Moran E, et al. Imaging amyloid deposition in Lewy body diseases. Neurology 2008;71(12):903–10.

103. Edison P, Rowe CC, Rinne JO, et al. Amyloid load in Parkinson's disease dementia and Lewy body dementia measured with [11C]PIB positron emission tomography. J Neurol Neurosurg Psychiatry 2008;79(12):1331–8.

Frontotemporal Lobar Degeneration: New Understanding Brings New Approaches

Maria Carmela Tartaglia, MD

KEYWORDS

- Frontotemporal dementia
- Semantic variant primary progressive aphasia
- Nonfluent variant primary progressive aphasia
- Frontotemporal lobar degeneration

Key Learning Points

1. Frontotemporal lobar degeneration (FTLD) is the pathologic term associated with several clinical syndromes.

2. Frontotemporal dementia (FTD) is a clinical term referring to behavioral variant FTD (bvFTD), nonfluent variant primary progressive aphasia (nfvPPA), and semantic variant primary progressive aphasia (svPPA)

3. Mutations in multiple genes cause FTLD.

4. Three different pathologic substrates can cause FTLD: tau, transactive DNA-binding protein 43 (TDP-43), and fused in sarcoma (FUS).

FTLD: A FAMILY OF SYNDROMES

FTLD is associated with several clinical syndromes involving behavior, language, and motor function. Until recently, the main syndromes encompassed by the clinical term FTD were bvFTD, nfvPPA, and svPPA. Recent discoveries revealed overlap at a clinical, genetic, and pathologic level between these syndromes and 3 other syndromes: FTD with motor neuron disease (FTD-MND), progressive supranuclear palsy (PSP), and corticobasal syndrome (CBS). The clinical expression of these syndromes is markedly different, reflecting selective injury of specific areas of the brain, which leads to the diverse signs and symptoms.[1]

Recent clinical-pathologic studies all emphasize that proper clinical assessments are paramount to clinicopathologic prediction.[2–4] Accurate diagnosis is the first step in the determination of the pathologic substrate because different syndromes are associated with different pathologies. In an effort to improve diagnosis, new criteria have been developed in the last year for bvFTD and the PPAs (semantic variant and nonfluent variant).[5,6]

bvFTD is characterized by dramatic personality and behavioral changes with prominent loss of social cognition.[7–11] New international research criteria have been established for bvFTD and focus on the behavioral/executive deficits (Box 1).[5]

As its name implies, bvFTD begins with prominent changes in social cognition, emotion, and behavior. Typical early symptoms include apathy, disinhibition, repetitive and compulsive behaviors, and progressive inability to represent the self and others, manifesting as shallow insight and lack of empathy. Disinhibition can lead to sociopathic behaviors such as being overly familiar with

---

Tanz Centre for Research in Neurodegenerative Diseases, University of Toronto, Tanz Building, 6 Queen's Park Cres West, Room 231, Toronto, ON, Canada M5S 3H2

E-mail address: ctartaglia@memory.ucsf.edu

Neuroimag Clin N Am 22 (2012) 83–97
doi:10.1016/j.nic.2011.11.009
1052-5149/12/$ – see front matter Crown Copyright © 2012 Published by Elsevier Inc. All rights reserved.

dress, and social style.[15] In bvFTD, overeating, weight gain, overstuffing the mouth, and idiosyncratic food fads occur.[16] Patients often display utilization behavior, manifested by grasping at items in view or repeatedly switching lights on and off.[12] Cognitive complaints, unlike in Alzheimer's disease (AD), are typically less dramatic than the behavioral changes, and the main deficits are in executive function.[9,11] bvFTD is the most common of the 3 main clinical subtypes of FTD, accounting for 56% of cases. It shows a male predominance (2:1), has the earliest age of onset (58 years at diagnosis), and progresses the most rapidly (3.4 years from diagnosis to death). bvFTD has the highest genetic susceptibility and is strongly associated with MND.[17,18]

nfvPPA (previously known as progressive nonfluent aphasia) is a disorder of expressive language and speech production.[11,19] New international criteria for PPA were recently published[6] and highlight the expressive language deficits with relative sparing of single sentence or word comprehension (**Boxes 2–4**). nfvPPA accounts for 25% of FTD and has an intermediate rate of progression (4.3 years from diagnosis) and genetic cause.[17] Nonfluent speech is often accompanied by agrammatism, phonemic paraphasias, anomia, and speech apraxia.[20] Speech is slow, effortful, and telegraphic, and in contrast to bvFTD, personal and interpersonal conduct, behavior, and insight are preserved early on.

svPPA, previously known as semantic dementia or temporal variant FTD, is a disorder with loss of semantic knowledge for words. It presents differently depending on which hemisphere is the site of pathology. Left-sided atrophy produces progressive loss of meaning for words, objects, and emotions.[11,19] In contrast, right-sided pathology is associated with behavioral changes. svPPA accounts for less than 20% of all FTD cases and shares an earlier age of onset with bvFTD but shows the slowest rate of progression (5.2 years from diagnosis to death).[17,18] svPPA has fewer cases of autosomal-dominant inheritance.

Although the term FTD was established to include only bvFTD, nfvPPA, and svPPA, it is now known that there are strong links and considerable overlap between FTD clinical syndromes and other conditions including PSP and CBS.[21] Many patients begin with an nfvPPA syndrome and later evolve into a clinical disorder suggestive of CBS or PSP.[22,23]

There are no consensus clinical research criteria for CBS but previous studies have described a progressive, asymmetric, akinetic-rigid syndrome that does not respond to levodopa treatment. Individuals have a combination of deficits

strangers, unsolicited sexual approaches, public urination, traffic violations, and shoplifting.[12–14] There can be dramatic personality changes, such as change in religious beliefs, political conviction,

Box 2
Inclusion and exclusion criteria for the diagnosis of PPA

Inclusion: criteria 1 to 3 must be answered positively

1. Most prominent clinical feature is difficulty with language (word-finding deficits, paraphasias, effortful speech, grammatical or comprehension deficits)

2. These deficits are the principal cause of impaired daily living activities (eg, problems with communication activity related to speech and language, such as using the telephone)

3. Aphasia should be the most prominent deficit for approximately 2 years since symptom onset.

Exclusion: criteria 1 to 4 must be answered negatively for a PPA diagnosis

1. Pattern of deficits is better accounted for by other nondegenerative nervous system or medical disorders (eg, neoplasm, cerebrovascular disease, hypothyroidism)

2. Cognitive disturbance is better accounted for by a psychiatric diagnosis (eg, depression, bipolar disorder, schizophrenia, preexisting personality disorder)

3. Prominent initial episodic memory, visual memory, and visuoperceptual impairments (eg, inability to copy simple line drawings)

4. Prominent initial behavioral disturbance (eg, marked disinhibition, emotional detachment, hyperorality, or repetitive/compulsive behaviors)

From Gorno-Tempini M, Hillis AE, Weintraub S, et al. Classification of primary progressive aphasia and its variants. Neurology 2011;76(11):1006–14.

Box 3
Diagnostic features for nfvPPA (also known as progressive nonfluent aphasia or PNFA, and as agrammatic PPA or PPA-G)

I. Clinical diagnosis of nfvPPA

At least one of the following core features must be present:

1. Grammatical errors and simplification in language production

2. Effortful, halting speech with inconsistent distortions, deletions, substitutions, insertions, or transpositions of speech sounds, particularly in polysyllabic words (often considered to reflect apraxia of speech)

At least 2 of the following 3 features must be present:

1. Impaired comprehension of syntactically complex sentences, with relatively spared comprehension of syntactically simpler sentences

2. Spared content, single-word comprehension

3. Spared object knowledge

II. Imaging-supported nfvPPA diagnosis

Both of the following criteria must be present:

1. Clinical diagnosis of nfvPPA

2. Imaging must show one or more of the following results:

   a. Predominant left posterior frontoinsular atrophy on magnetic resonance (MR) imaging

   b. Predominant left posterior frontoinsular hypoperfusion or hypometabolism on single-photon emission computed tomography (SPECT) or positron emission tomography (PET)

III. nfvPPA with definite pathology

Clinical diagnosis (criterion 1) and either criterion 2 or 3 must be present:

1. Clinical diagnosis of nfvPPA

2. Histopathologic evidence of a specific pathology (eg, FTLD-tau, FTLD-TDP) on biopsy or post mortem

3. Presence of a known pathogenic mutation

attributable to cortical dysfunction, such as apraxia, language difficulties, and cortical sensory loss or neglect as well as symptoms attributable to basal ganglia dysfunction such as rigidity or dystonia.[24] Cognitively, planning and other aspects of executive function are impaired in CBS.[25] In October 2009, a group of corticobasal degeneration (CBD)/CBS researchers met to determine consensus clinical research criteria for CBS. The new criteria (Litvan and colleagues, manuscript in preparation) will be similar to the previous criteria but will also include dementia syndromes that have been associated with CBD.

Consensus research criteria have been developed for PSP and have been reported to have excellent predictive power for underlying PSP pathology.[26,27] PSP is named for its characteristic eye movement abnormalities, and a diagnosis of probable PSP requires a slowly progressive disorder with onset after age 40 years and a vertical supranuclear gaze palsy of eye movements and falls within the first year of diagnosis.

Box 4

Diagnostic criteria for svPPA (also known as semantic dementia or PPA-S)

I. Clinical diagnosis of svPPA

Both of the following core features must be present:

1. Poor confrontation naming (of pictures or objects), particularly for low familiarity or low frequency items
2. Impaired single-word comprehension

At least 3 of the following other diagnostic features must be present:

1. Poor object or person knowledge, particularly for low frequency or low familiarity items
2. Surface dyslexia or dysgraphia
3. Spared repetition
4. Spared motor speech

II. Imaging-supported svPPA diagnosis

Both of the following criteria must be present:

1. Clinical diagnosis of svPPA
2. Imaging must show one or more of the following results:
   a. Predominant anterior temporal lobe atrophy
   b. Predominant anterior temporal hypoperfusion or hypometabolism on SPECT or PET

III. svPPA with definite pathology

Clinical diagnosis (criterion 1) and either criterion 2 or 3 must be present:

1. Clinical diagnosis of svPPA
2. Histopathologic evidence of a specific pathology (eg, FTLD-tau, FTLD-TDP) on biopsy or post mortem
3. Presence of a known pathogenic mutation

Other supportive criteria include prominent axial rigidity, early dysphagia and dysarthria, apathy, and cognitive impairments consisting mainly of executive dysfunction. Significant behavioral changes including impulsivity, perseveration, and diminished judgment also feature in PSP.

MND may co-occur with bvFTD-like symptoms, or, less commonly, with svPPA or nfvPPA,[28,29] and the term FTD-MND has been applied to these cases. FTD-MND most commonly affects lower motor neurons to the bulbar and upper limb musculature. The close relationship between dementia and MND (also known as amyotrophic lateral sclerosis) surfaced with the discovery of overlapping genetics,[30] including a recent discovery that the expanded hexanucleotide repeat in a noncoding region of chromosome 9 is associated with MND and FTD.[31,32] In addition, common neuropathologic substrates exist between the 2 syndromes,[33] suggesting a strong connection between them. In prospective studies, up to 50% of patients with FTD had possible or probable MND,[28] and 50% of patients with MND who underwent behavioral and neuropsychological evaluation had measurable (mainly frontal/executive and behavioral) cognitive deficits, and many met criteria for an FTD syndrome.[34]

FTLD: UNDERSTANDING THE SYNDROME-PATHOLOGY RELATIONSHIP

The underlying pathology of FTLD has proved more complex than anticipated. It is now known that at least 3 different molecular pathologies exist consisting of abnormal protein aggregation: tau, TDP-43, and FUS.

Abnormal tau deposition or aggregation was the first pathologic substrate described and, until recently, it was believed to be the main cause of FTLD. Tau is a protein that binds to and stabilizes microtubules that are necessary for maintaining neuronal shape and for transport of cellular cargo.[35] The abnormal tau can be seen in neurons, glia, or both. The syndromes that associate with abnormal tau deposition are known as tauopathies. PSP is associated exclusively with tau pathology, whereas in the case of CBS, although most cases are caused by abnormal tau aggregation, there is recognition that other diseases can cause the syndrome such as TDP-43 or AD. Nonfluent variant PPA is also primarily a tauopathy but can also be associated with TDP-43 or AD. A variety of mutations have been identified in the microtubule-associated protein tau (MAPT) gene that lead to bvFTD, nfvPPA, PSP, and CBS.[36]

Tau-negative cases of FTLD stain for ubiquitin, an integral part of the degradative system.[37] Most ubiquitin-positive inclusions observed in FTLD result from the accumulation of inclusions that stain for TDP-43, a widely expressed nuclear protein with presumed functions in transcription regulation and exon skipping.[38] These neuronal or cytoplasmic ubiquitinated inclusions are usually seen in affected cortex, dentate granule cells,[39] and primary motor cortex, spinal cord, or brain stem motor neurons in FTD-MND.[40]

Four distinct patterns of pathologic features and regional variability were observed in cases of TDP-43 proteinopathy,[41–43] and these patterns have clinical relevance, because they are specific to some, although not all, of the syndromes.[44] FTLD-TDP A, which features many neuronal cytoplasmic inclusions and short dystrophic neurites in layer 2 of the cortex, is seen in bvFTD, nfvPPA, and nearly all patients with granulin (GRN) mutations.[45] Patients with FTLD-TDP and a GRN polymorphism of the T-allele of rs5848 often show an FTLD-TDP A pathologic pattern.[46] FTLD-TDP B is transcortical and features some neuronal cytoplasmic inclusions and few dystrophic neurites and is seen in bvFTD and FTD-MND. FTLD-TDP C is also predominantly in layer 2, features many, long, dystrophic neurites and few neuronal cytoplasmic inclusions, and is seen in svPPA and bvFTD. A fourth subtype, FTLD-TDP D, is seen only in valosin-containing protein (VCP) mutations and consists of many short dystrophic neurites, many lentiform neuronal intranuclear inclusions, and few neuronal cytoplasmic inclusions. The pathology are seen in all layers. The clinical phenotype associated with the VCP mutations is inclusion body myopathy with Paget disease of bone and FTD.

The inclusions in ubiquitin-positive, TDP-43–negative cases of FTLD were recently discovered to stain for the FUS protein. FUS is a ubiquitously expressed DNA/RNA-binding protein involved in multiple aspects of gene expression, transcription regulation, RNA splicing, transport, and translation.[47] FUS pathology is reportedly associated with a distinct clinical phenotype that includes young onset, prominent obsessionality, repetitive behaviors and rituals, social withdrawal and lack of engagement, hyperorality with pica, and marked stimulus-bound behavior including use behavior.[48,49] In addition, FUS cases show severe caudate atrophy. This pathologic subtype may be the easiest to disentangle from the other FTLD pathologic substrates.

Clinicopathologic correlations have shown that certain FTLD syndromes are reliably associated with specific proteinopathies: FTD-MND is associated almost uniquely with FTLD-TDP, with only a few cases ascribed to FUS. svPPA also is almost always associated with FTLD-TDP, with only rare cases of FTLD-tau described. PSP is exclusively a tauopathy.[2–4] However, the rest of the syndromes are difficult to predict because nfvPPA is most often associated with a tauopathy,[50] but FTLD-TDP and AD pathology can cause this clinical syndrome in some cases.[2–4] bvFTD is difficult to predict, because it can be associated with FTLD-tau, FTLD-TDP, FTLD-FUS, or AD. CBS is similarly difficult to predict, because although most cases are associated with FTLD-tau, there are reports of FTLD-TDP and AD as the pathologic substrate of CBS.[2–4,51,52]

GENETICS OF FTLD

Although most FTLD cases are sporadic, unlike the other dementing illnesses, FTLD has a strong familial component because up to 40% to 50% of cases are diagnosed as familial and 10% show an autosomal-dominant pattern of inheritance.[53] Multiple genes have been implicated in FTLD, including MAPT (chromosome 17), GRN (chromosome 17), VCP (chromosome 9), chromatin-modifying protein 2B (also known as charged multivesicular body protein 2B gene) CHMP2B (chromosome 3), and FUS gene (chromosome 16).[54–56] Recently, a novel mutation has been discovered as the most common cause of familial FTD and MND; it consists of an expanded hexanucleotide repeat in a noncoding region of chromosome 9 open reading frame 72.[31,32] The gene encodes an uncharacterized protein with no known domains or function, but which is highly conserved across species.

These genetic abnormalities are associated with specific proteinopathies so that MAPT mutation leads to a tauopathy, VCP and GRN mutations and expanded hexanucleotide repeat to TDP-43 proteinopathy, and FUS mutation to a FUSopathy.[38,47] The abnormal protein in CMP2B mutations remains elusive to date; no specific protein has been discovered to identify the inclusions.

FTLD was first linked to chromosome 17 (MAPT gene) by Wilhelmsen and colleagues.[54] MAPT mutations are associated with tau pathology, and more than 40 different mutations in the MAPT gene have been reported in association with familial FTD syndromes.[57] Humans carry an equal ratio of 3R and 4R tau, but mutations in the tau intron lead to increases in the ratio of 4R to 3R tau. A wide spectrum of disorders has been reported with tau inclusions, including bvFTD, nfvPPA, CBD, and PSP.[58]

Although MAPT mutations were the first discovered, epidemiologic studies have identified GRN mutations in 5% to 11% of all FTD and 11% to 26% of patients with a family history,[59] making it the most common cause of genetic FTLD. This mutation is also on chromosome 17 but at 17q21 in the progranulin (GRN) gene.[60] More than 50 progranulin mutations have been found since it was discovered in 2006,[57] and these mutations lead to deficient protein levels of progranulin.[60] The role of progranulin in neurodegeneration is still unknown, although progranulin is a trophic factor, and is implicated in wound healing, tumor growth, inflammation, and brain development in mice; it promotes neuronal survival and stimulates neuritic outgrowth in cultures of rat motor and cortical neurons.[61] Progranulin mutations are associated with phenotypic heterogeneity, even within family members with the same mutation. bvFTD is the most common presentation of GRN mutation followed by nfvPPA and svPPA although parkinsonian and AD syndromes are also seen.[57] The ubiquitinated inclusions associated with progranulin mutations stain for TDP-43.[38]

The likelihood of a genetic mutation associated with the FTLD syndrome varies across the different subtypes. bvFTD and FTD-MND are the most strongly familial of the FTLD syndromes. Semantic variant is the least familial, whereas nfvPPA lies in between bvFTD and svPPA.[62] As a risk for FTD, the role of apolipoprotein E4 seems to be small,[63] although E4 may expand the pathologic damage in frontal regions in FTD.[64]

Polymorphisms, in the absence of mutation, have gained attention as possible contributors to pathology. Rademakers and colleagues[46] showed a significant reduction in progranulin protein level in homozygous GRN T-allele carriers in vivo, and the neuropathology of homozygous GRN rs5848 T-allele carriers frequently resembled the pathologic FTLD-ubiquitin subtype of GRN mutation carriers. Structural differences in brain areas important for social cognition (ie, left medial orbital white matter [WM], right fusiform WM, and right supramarginal total volume) were observed between normal controls with homozygous T-alleles of a common genetic variant rs5848 in the GRN gene compared with the CT and CC polymorphisms.[65] The MAPT H1H1 haplotype is overly represented in patients with CBS and PSP; healthy white controls show between 60% and 70% homozygosity for H1, approximately 90% of patients with CBS and PSP are H1H1.[66] How polymorphisms interact with the molecular pathology to determine the specific pathology as well as its distribution is unknown.

The ubiquitinated inclusions associated with progranulin mutations stain not for progranulin but instead for TDP-43.[38,60] In contrast to sporadic cases of FTD with ubiquitin-TDP-43 pathology, in which the inclusions occur in the cytoplasm, with progranulin mutations, TDP-43 is found in the nucleus. This naturally occurring protein is found in the nucleus and is implicated in exon skipping and transcription regulation.[47] Mutations in the TARDBP-43 gene localized on chromosome 1 have recently been identified in a few families with autosomal-dominant MND,[38,67] which supports the role of TDP-43 in the pathophysiology of MND.

IMAGING FTLD AND THE PATHOLOGIC SUBSTRATES

The FTLD syndromes share similar pathologic substrates but their clinical expression is markedly different and reflects selective injury of certain areas of the brain, which leads to the diverse signs and symptoms.[1] Specific atrophy patterns evident on structural images have been the basis of much of the current research in FTD,[68–71] and recent research shows that imaging has prognostic implications.[72] bvFTD is associated with loss of gray matter (GM) in the frontal and temporal lobes and in particular the ventromedial frontal cortex, the posterior orbital frontal regions, the insula bilaterally, and the anterior cingulate cortex (ACC) (Fig. 1).[68] These regions are components of the emotional processing systems of the brain,[73] so that their involvement in FTD explains the unique behavioral symptoms seen in that disorder.[74–77] Relationships have been established between regional brain abnormalities and specific clinical features such as social and emotional processing,[74–78] social cognition,[76,78] emotion processing,[79] frontal/executive functions,[80] grammatical and semantic processing,[81,82] and self-awareness.[83] svPPA shows progressive anterior temporal atrophy (Fig. 2A and B).[84] Left-predominant cases present as a fluent, anomic aphasia,[85] whereas patients with predominantly right anterior temporal atrophy present with a behavioral syndrome characterized by a flat affect, emotional blunting, and alterations in social conduct plus deficits in empathy and inability to recognize people's emotions.[86] nfvPPA, a disorder of expressive language and speech production, is characterized anatomically by left perisylvian atrophy, in particular, atrophy of the left frontal operculum (see Fig. 2C).[11] CBS is characterized by frontoparietal atrophy[87] and PSP shows early midbrain tectum atrophy.[88]

The syndrome-specific atrophy patterns are useful for diagnosing the different syndromes, and there is increasing evidence that they may be of use in differentiating FTLD-tau from FTLD-TDP. Focusing on patients with GRN or tau mutations, and associated TDP-43 and tau pathology, respectively, 2 independent studies have shown different atrophy patterns amongst the 2 groups of mutation carriers. Patients with GRN mutations (TDP-43 pathology) showed asymmetric atrophy of frontal, insular, cingulate, parietal, and temporal areas linked by intrahemispheric long association tracts. Patients with MAPT mutations (tau pathology), alternatively, were associated with more restricted but bihemispheric atrophy of anteromedial temporal and orbitofrontal areas linked via the fornices and uncinate fasciculi.[89] Similar, although not identical, results had been previously reported with patients with GRN mutations showing GM loss in posterior temporal and parietal lobes and patients with MAPT mutations

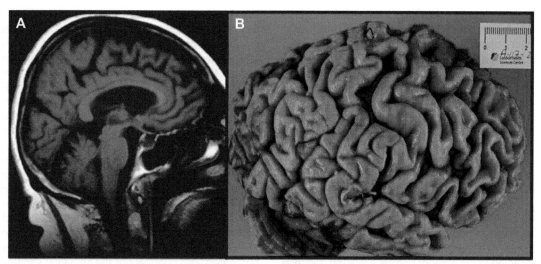

Fig. 1. View of a patient with bvFTD showing a unique pattern of brain atrophy in the ventromedial frontal cortex, the posterior orbital frontal regions, the insula, and the ACC. Notice the anterior atrophy with relative sparing of parietal and occipital regions. (A) Midsagittal T1-weighted MR imaging of patient with bvFTD. (B) Post-mortem specimen of patient with bvFTD. Notice the anterior atrophy compared with the preserved posterior part of the brain.

showing anteromedial temporal lobe atrophy.[90] When compared directly, the individuals with MAPT mutation showed greater GM loss in the medial temporal lobes, insula, and putamen than the individuals with GRN mutation. Another study looked at FTLD-TDP subtypes specifically and revealed differing imaging characteristics based on subtype: FTLD-TDP A (nfvPPA and CBS) with asymmetric atrophy (either left-predominant or right-predominant) involving more dorsal areas including frontal, temporal, and inferior parietal cortices as well as striatum and thalamus; FTLD-TDP B (bvFTD and FTD-MND) with relatively symmetric atrophy of the medial temporal, medial prefrontal, and orbitofrontal-insular cortices; and FTLD-TDP C (svPPA) was associated with asymmetric anterior temporal lobe atrophy (either left-predominant or right-predominant) as well as orbitofrontal lobes and insulae.[91]

The focus of research in FTLD and AD has been GM pathology, although WM injury has been observed pathologically, because FTLD-tau, FTLD-TDP, and FTLD-FUS all show WM pathology.[56,92–95] In FTLD-TDP, glial cytoplasmic inclusions and rare threadlike inclusions were found throughout the frontal and temporal lobes.[92] Based on morphology and double-labeling experiments, these investigators hypothesized that the affected glial cells most likely represent oligodendrocytes. PSP and CBD (a pathologic term for underlying pathology of most CBS) are classic tauopathies, and are now part of the FTLD spectrum; both show extensive glial pathology in the WM.[96,97] Significant WM pathology has also been reported in Pick disease, and in some areas was more extensive than in the adjacent GM.[93]

Structural imaging has shown reduced left frontal WM volume in patients with FTD compared

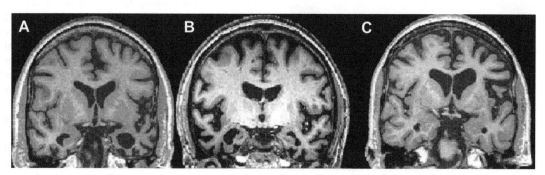

Fig. 2. Coronal view of patient with svPPA showing significant (A) left and (B) right temporal atrophy. (C) Coronal view of patient with nonfluent variant of FTD, showing significant left insular atrophy.

with controls.[98] Diffusion tensor imaging (DTI) informs on the integrity of WM by providing different metrics related to the diffusivity of water: axial diffusivity is parallel to the axonal direction and alterations are believed to reflect primarily axonal injury; radial diffusivity is perpendicular to the axon and believed to relate primarily to myelin damage.[99,100] The axial and radial parameters can be averaged to provide a mean diffusivity (MD) and can be used to compute the fractional anisotropy (FA).[101] One of the advantages of DTI is that it is possible to investigate specific WM tracts such as the uncinate fasciculus (Unc) (Fig. 3) and even segregate out subcomponents of complex tracts like the superior longitudinal fasciculus (SLF) (Fig. 4). Comparing bvFTD and AD with normal controls and each other, reduced FA was observed in the anterior corpus callosum, bilateral anterior and descending cingulum (Cg) tracts, and Unc in patients with bvFTD compared with normal age-matched controls and in the anterior corpus callosum and bilateral Unc fasciculus compared with patients with AD.[102] Patients with AD also showed areas of decreased FA compared with controls but in a more restricted fashion and they showed no areas of worse damage when compared with bvFTD.

A DTI study evaluated WM alterations in specific tracts in patients with PPA and found striking differences according to the clinical syndrome. In nfvPPA, focal injury was observed in the SLF and when looking closely at all the subcomponents of the SLF, all subcomponents were affected.[103] Patients with semantic variant showed severe involvement of the Unc bilaterally and the anterior portion of the inferior longitudinal fasciculus (ILF).

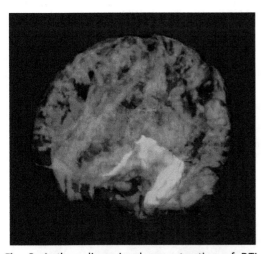

Fig. 3. A three-dimensional reconstruction of DTI-derived uncinate in normal controls. (*Courtesy of* S. Galantucci.)

The logopenic patients showed the most consistent DTI changes in the left temporoparietal component of the SLF. These findings are important for clinical expression of these PPA variants and so the dorsal network injury in nfvPPA may be partially responsible for the motor speech difficulties and agrammatism typical of this variant, whereas a dysfunction of the ventral language system accounts for the typical combination of impaired semantics and spared phonology, grammar, and fluency language domains in svPPA. In logopenic patients, tracts important for sentence repetition and phonological short-term memory are most injured.[104] Furthermore, nonfluent and semantic variants showed different patterns of alterations in their DTI metrics. The nfvPPA was sparing of their axial diffusivity compared with controls but the semantic variants had significantly different FA, MD, axial, and radial diffusivity compared with controls, suggesting that the svPPA may have both axonal and myelin damage; in the nonfluent variant, the pathology may be restricted to the myelin.[104]

In an effort to try to understand the contribution of WM tract injury to some of the cognitive and behavioral deficits observed in FTLD, several studies have included both GM and WM metrics. A look at executive dysfunction in bvFTD revealed the left anterior Cg tract to be a significant predictor of executive impairments, even after correcting for GM volumes adjacent to the tract.[105] A recent study examining syntax in patients with PPA showed that the arcuate fasciculus/SLF correlated significantly with syntax production and comprehension and not with semantic function, whereas the extreme capsule fiber system, a more recently describe WM tract, which connects the frontal operculum to midposterior temporal cortex, was predictive of lexical processing but not syntax (Fig. 5).[106]

We have used DTI and GM volumetrics to assess the relative contribution of WM and GM injury to social cognitive dysfunction in PPA.[107] We found a relationship between emotion detection and WM tract integrity in bilateral Unc and bilateral anterior ILF in addition to the bilateral orbitofrontal GM, and bilateral anterior temporal lobe GM. Certain personality traits like coldness correlated with WM tract injury in right anterior ILF, right Unc, and right arcuate in addition to GM in the anterior temporal, posterior temporal, and orbitofrontal cortex. Overall, these results suggest that WM connections in right anterior temporal and ventromedial frontal regions may also be important for emotional sensitivity and expressiveness, in addition to the known GM-personality relationships in these regions.

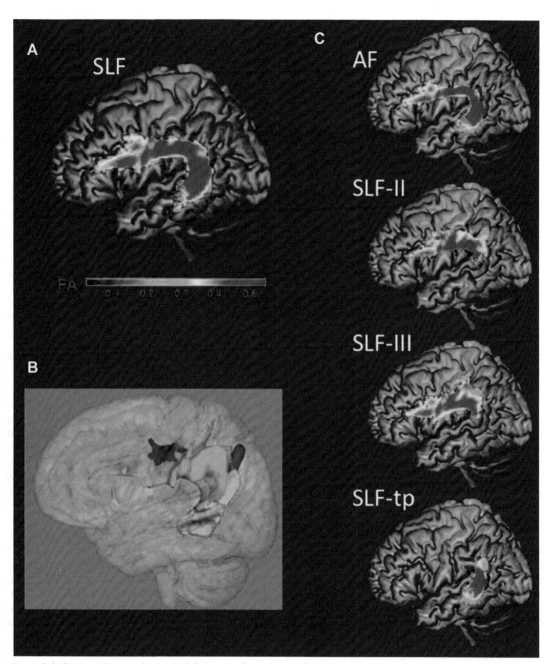

Fig. 4. (*A*) The FA values in the probability maps for SLF in healthy controls generated with FSL and overlayed on a standard MNI brain. The chromatic scale represents average FA values ranging from lower (*violet-blue*) to higher (*yellow-red*) values. (*B*) A three-dimensional reconstruction of SLF with subcomponents: arcuate fasciculus (AF) (*blue*), SLF II (angular gyrus to frontal operculum) (*green*), SLF III (supramarginal gyrus to frontal operculum) (*red*), SLF temporoparietal component (*yellow*). (*C*) FA maps SLF subcomponents in healthy controls.

As other imaging modalities emerge, they provide unique, novel information on different facets of FTLD. Until recently, little thought had been given to neurodegenerative diseases causing a network malfunction. Resting-state functional MR imaging has been used to elucidate coherent large-scale brain networks subserving vision, auditory function, language, and attention, and a frontal opercular network that has been related to stimulus salience.[108–110] These data are acquired by having patients undergo task-free (or resting-state) MR imaging to identify the structures in which a blood oxygen level-dependent signal shows intercorrelated fluctuations in functionally

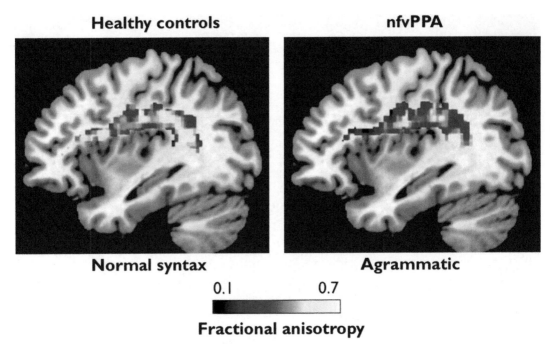

Fractional anisotropy

Fig. 5. FA maps of the left SLF in normal controls and nfvPPA. Lower FA in SLF of individuals with nfvPPA who are agrammatic. (*Courtesy of* S. Wilson.)

connected networks over time.[111] This approach has revealed a set of highly reproducible intrinsic connectivity networks recruiting multiple structures into a coordinated effort to perform a generalized cognitive function. The networks derived from the resting-state method closely match task-evoked functional MR imaging patterns[110] and DTI analysis in humans confirms that these networks closely reflect structural connectivity.[112] In FTD, a salience network that includes the dorsal anterior cingulate and orbital/frontoinsular regions, and tracks with emotional measures, has shown alterations.[109]

Arterial spin labeling (ASL) measures brain perfusion entirely noninvasively.[113] This measurement is accomplished by using the physical principles of MR imaging to magnetically label blood water as an endogenous tracer for blood flow. ASL-MR imaging can readily be performed in the same scan session as structural MR imaging. Its use in FTD is just emerging and discordant GM atrophy without hypoperfusion was observed in the premotor cortex in FTD, whereas concordant GM atrophy and hypoperfusion were observed in the right prefrontal cortex and bilateral medial frontal lobe.[114] These patterns may be important for function and require histopathologic correlation.

Functional imaging and ligand-based imaging have provided some insight into the pathophysiology of FTLD. PET is most often used with [18F]fluorodeoxyglucose to measure brain energy metabolism. In FTD, hypometabolism is observed in the frontal and anterior temporal regions, with relative sparing of posterior brain regions. Amyloid imaging is usually negative in FTLD and so is useful for excluding AD as the underlying pathology.[115]

SUMMARY

FTLD is at the center of a paradigm shift: for the first time, disease-modifying treatments are becoming a reality. In a field that had little to offer its patients, in terms of disease modification, there are now clinical trials of protein-specific treatments. The need for pathologic as well as clinical diagnosis has never been so essential as it is today. Treatment of neurodegenerative disease requires early pathologic diagnosis because reversal of disease is unlikely. Multimodal assessments for pathologic diagnosis will likely emerge as critically important for the care of patients. The future of treatment in FTLD will begin with accurate clinical assessment, brain imaging that will likely involve combinations of imaging techniques to identify the presence of a molecular abnormality, and a protein-specific treatment that can potentially halt the disease, or at least delay progression.

SUMMARY CONCEPTS

1. FTD is a clinical term that encompasses a heterogeneous group of patients who share focal degeneration within the anterior frontal, temporal, and insular regions. This term includes bvFTD, nfvPPA, and svPPA.

2. FTLD is the pathologic term that encompasses several syndromes that involve focal atrophy. Recently, the discovery of overlapping genetics and disease has led to the incorporation of 3 other clinical phenotypes under this rubric so that now, in addition to bvFTD, nfvPPA, and svPPA, PSP, CBD, and FTD with MND have been added.

3. bvFTD is associated with an early change in personality and behavior. bvFTD is associated with GM atrophy in the frontal and temporal lobes, in particular the ventromedial frontal cortex, the posterior orbital frontal regions, the insula bilaterally, and the ACC.

4. nfvPPA presents with nonfluent speech and language. nfvPPA is characterized anatomically by left perisylvian atrophy, in particular, atrophy of the left frontal operculum (Broca areas 44, 45, and 47).

5. svPPA is a disorder of semantic knowledge for words. svPPA shows progressive anterior temporal atrophy with the clinical syndrome determined by the side of the brain with the greatest atrophy. Left-predominant cases present as a fluent, anomic aphasia, whereas right anterior temporal atrophy presents with a behavioral syndrome characterized by a flat affect, emotional blunting, and alterations in social conduct plus deficits in empathy and inability to recognize people's emotions.

6. FTD is the second most common dementia in those less than 65 years of age; it accounts for 5% to 6% of all dementias and is responsible for up to 17% of early-onset (<70 years) dementias in autopsy series.

7. FTLD can be classified into 2 main pathologic subtypes based on the pattern of neuronal and glial inclusion: (1) tau-positive lesions with tau-positive inclusions (Pick disease, CBD, PSP) and (2) tau-negative, ubiquitin-positive inclusions, including TDP-43 and FUS.

8. GM and WM pathology contribute to some of the deficits seen in FTLD.

9. GM and WM pathology can be evaluated in vivo using MR imaging.

REFERENCES

1. Brun A. Frontal lobe degeneration of non-Alzheimer type revisited. Dementia 1993;4:126–31.

2. Snowden JS, Thompson JC, Stopford CL, et al. The clinical diagnosis of early-onset dementias: diagnostic accuracy and clinicopathological relationships. Brain 2011;134(Pt 9):2478–92.

3. Josephs KA, Hodges JR, Snowden JS, et al. Neuropathological background of phenotypical variability in frontotemporal dementia. Acta Neuropathol 2011;122:137–53.

4. Rohrer J, Lashley T, Schott J, et al. Clinical and neuroanatomical signatures of tissue pathology in frontotemporal lobar degeneration. Brain 2011; 134(Pt 9):2565–81.

5. Rascovsky K, Hodges JR, Knopman D, et al. Sensitivity of revised diagnostic criteria for the behavioural variant of frontotemporal dementia. Brain 2011; 134(Pt 9):2456–77.

6. Gorno-Tempini M, Hillis AE, Weintraub S, et al. Classification of primary progressive aphasia and its variants. Neurology 2011;76(11):1006–14.

7. Gustafson L. Frontal lobe degeneration of non-Alzheimer type. II. Clinical picture and differential diagnosis. Arch Gerontol Geriatr 1987;6:209–23.

8. Neary D, Snowden JS, Northen B, et al. Dementia of frontal lobe type. J Neurol Neurosurg Psychiatry 1988;51:353–61.

9. Miller BL, Cummings JL, Villanueva-Meyer J, et al. Frontal lobe degeneration: clinical, neuropsychological, and SPECT characteristics. Neurology 1991;41:1374–82.

10. The Lund and Manchester Groups. Clinical and neuropathological criteria for frontotemporal dementia. J Neurol Neurosurg Psychiatry 1994; 57:416–8.

11. Neary D, Snowden JS, Gustafson L, et al. Frontotemporal lobar degeneration: a consensus on clinical diagnostic criteria. Neurology 1998;51:1546–54.

12. Gustafson L. Clinical picture of frontal lobe degeneration of non-Alzheimer type. Dementia 1993;4:143–8.

13. Miller BL, Darby A, Benson DF, et al. Aggressive, socially disruptive and antisocial behaviour associated with fronto-temporal dementia. Br J Psychiatry 1997;170:150–4.

14. Mendez MF, Chen AK, Shapira JS, et al. Acquired sociopathy and frontotemporal dementia. Dement Geriatr Cogn Disord 2005;20:99–104.

15. Miller BL, Seeley WW, Mychack P, et al. Neuroanatomy of the self: evidence from patients with frontotemporal dementia. Neurology 2001;57:817–21.

16. Miller BL, Darby AL, Swartz JR, et al. Dietary changes, compulsions and sexual behavior in frontotemporal degeneration. Dementia 1995;6:195–9.

17. Johnson JK, Diehl J, Mendez MF, et al. Frontotemporal lobar degeneration: demographic characteristics of 353 patients. Arch Neurol 2005;62:925–30.

18. Roberson ED, Hesse JH, Rose KD, et al. Frontotemporal dementia progresses to death faster than Alzheimer disease. Neurology 2005;65:719–25.

19. Hodges JR, Miller B. The classification, genetics and neuropathology of frontotemporal dementia. Introduction to the special topic papers: part I. Neurocase 2001;7:31–5.

20. Gorno-Tempini ML, Ogar JM, Brambati SM, et al. Anatomical correlates of early mutism in progressive nonfluent aphasia. Neurology 2006;67:1849–51.

21. Boeve BF, Lang AE, Litvan I. Corticobasal degeneration and its relationship to progressive supranuclear palsy and frontotemporal dementia. Ann Neurol 2003;54(Suppl 5):S15–9.

22. Gorno-Tempini ML, Dronkers NF, Rankin KP, et al. Cognition and anatomy in three variants of primary progressive aphasia. Ann Neurol 2004;55:335–46.

23. Josephs KA, Petersen RC, Knopman DS, et al. Clinicopathologic analysis of frontotemporal and corticobasal degenerations and PSP. Neurology 2006;66:41–8.

24. Litvan I, Bhatia KP, Burn DJ, et al. Movement Disorders Society Scientific Issues Committee report: SIC Task Force appraisal of clinical diagnostic criteria for Parkinsonian disorders. Mov Disord 2003;18:467–86.

25. Murray R, Neumann M, Forman MS, et al. Cognitive and motor assessment in autopsy-proven corticobasal degeneration. Neurology 2007;68:1274–83.

26. Litvan I, Agid Y, Calne D, et al. Clinical research criteria for the diagnosis of progressive supranuclear palsy (Steele-Richardson-Olszewski syndrome): report of the NINDS-SPSP international workshop. Neurology 1996;47:1–9.

27. Litvan I, Agid Y, Jankovic J, et al. Accuracy of clinical criteria for the diagnosis of progressive supranuclear palsy (Steele-Richardson-Olszewski syndrome). Neurology 1996;46:922–30.

28. Lomen-Hoerth C, Anderson T, Miller B. The overlap of amyotrophic lateral sclerosis and frontotemporal dementia. Neurology 2002;59:1077–9.

29. Lomen-Hoerth C, Murphy J, Langmore S, et al. Are amyotrophic lateral sclerosis patients cognitively normal? Neurology 2003;60:1094–7.

30. Foster NL, Wilhelmsen K, Sima AA, et al. Frontotemporal dementia and parkinsonism linked to chromosome 17: a consensus conference. Conference Participants. Ann Neurol 1997;41:706–15.

31. Renton AE, Waite A, Simón-Sánchez J, et al. A hexanucleotide repeat expansion in C9ORF72 is the cause of chromosome 9p21-linked ALS-FTD. Neuron 2011;72(2):257–68.

32. DeJesus-Hernandez M, Boeve BF, Boxer AL, et al. Expanded GGGGCC hexanucleotide repeat in noncoding region of C9ORF72 causes chromosome 9p-Linked FTD and ALS. Neuron 2011;72(2):245–56.

33. Cooper PN, Jackson M, Lennox G, et al. Tau, ubiquitin, and alpha B-crystallin immunohistochemistry define the principal causes of degenerative frontotemporal dementia. Arch Neurol 1995;52:1011–5.

34. Strong MJ, Lomen-Hoerth C, Caselli RJ, et al. Cognitive impairment, frontotemporal dementia, and the motor neuron diseases. Ann Neurol 2003;54(Suppl 5):S20–3.

35. Brunden KR, Trojanowski JQ, Lee VM. Advances in tau-focused drug discovery for Alzheimer's disease and related tauopathies. Nat Rev Drug Discov 2009;8:783–93.

36. Kertesz A. Pick's complex and FTDP-17. Mov Disord 2003;18(Suppl 6):S57–62.

37. Tai HC, Schuman EM. Ubiquitin, the proteasome and protein degradation in neuronal function and dysfunction. Nat Rev Neurosci 2008;9:826–38.

38. Neumann M, Sampathu DM, Kwong LK, et al. Ubiquitinated TDP-43 in frontotemporal lobar degeneration and amyotrophic lateral sclerosis. Science 2006;314:130–3.

39. Josephs KA, Holton JL, Rossor MN, et al. Frontotemporal lobar degeneration and ubiquitin immunohistochemistry. Neuropathol Appl Neurobiol 2004;30:369–73.

40. Bigio EH, Lipton AM, White CL 3rd, et al. Frontotemporal and motor neurone degeneration with neurofilament inclusion bodies: additional evidence for overlap between FTD and ALS. Neuropathol Appl Neurobiol 2003;29:239–53.

41. Mackenzie IR, Baborie A, Pickering-Brown S, et al. Heterogeneity of ubiquitin pathology in frontotemporal lobar degeneration: classification and relation to clinical phenotype. Acta Neuropathol 2006;112:539–49.

42. Sampathu DM, Neumann M, Kwong LK, et al. Pathological heterogeneity of frontotemporal lobar degeneration with ubiquitin-positive inclusions delineated by ubiquitin immunohistochemistry and novel monoclonal antibodies. Am J Pathol 2006;169:1343–52.

43. Mackenzie IR, Neumann M, Baborie A, et al. A harmonized classification system for FTLD-TDP pathology. Acta Neuropathol 2011;122:111–3.

44. Cairns NJ, Neumann M, Bigio EH, et al. TDP-43 in familial and sporadic frontotemporal lobar degeneration with ubiquitin inclusions. Am J Pathol 2007;171:227–40.

45. Mackenzie IR, Baker M, Pickering-Brown S, et al. The neuropathology of frontotemporal lobar degeneration caused by mutations in the progranulin gene. Brain 2006;129:3081–90.

46. Rademakers R, Eriksen JL, Baker M, et al. Common variation in the miR-659 binding-site of GRN is a major risk factor for TDP43-positive frontotemporal dementia. Hum Mol Genet 2008;17:3631–42.

47. Buratti E, Baralle FE. Multiple roles of TDP-43 in gene expression, splicing regulation, and human disease. Front Biosci 2008;13:867–78.

48. Rohrer JD, Lashley T, Holton J, et al. The clinical and neuroanatomical phenotype of FUS associated frontotemporal lobar degeneration. J Neurol Neurosurg Psychiatry 2011;82(12):1405–7.

49. Snowden JS, Hu Q, Rollinson S, et al. The most common type of FTLD-FUS (aFTLD-U) is associated with a distinct clinical form of frontotemporal dementia but is not related to mutations in the FUS gene. Acta Neuropathol 2011;122:99–110.

50. Grossman M. Primary progressive aphasia: clinicopathological correlations. Nat Rev Neurol 2010;6:88–97.

51. Neumann M, Tolnay M, Mackenzie IR. The molecular basis of frontotemporal dementia. Expert Rev Mol Med 2009;11:e23.

52. Tartaglia MC, Sidhu M, Laluz V, et al. Sporadic corticobasal syndrome due to FTLD-TDP. Acta Neuropathol 2009;119:365–74.

53. Seelaar H, Kamphorst W, Rosso SM, et al. Distinct genetic forms of frontotemporal dementia. Neurology 2008;71:1220–6.

54. Wilhelmsen KC, Lynch T, Pavlou E, et al. Localization of disinhibition-dementia-parkinsonism-amyotrophy complex to 17q21-22. Am J Hum Genet 1994;55:1159–65.

55. Bigio EH. Update on recent molecular and genetic advances in frontotemporal lobar degeneration. J Neuropathol Exp Neurol 2008;67:635–48.

56. Neumann M, Rademakers R, Roeber S, et al. A new subtype of frontotemporal lobar degeneration with FUS pathology. Brain 2009;132:2922–31.

57. Rademakers R, Hutton M. The genetics of frontotemporal lobar degeneration. Curr Neurol Neurosci Rep 2007;7:434–42.

58. Bugiani O. The many ways to frontotemporal degeneration and beyond. Neurol Sci 2007;28:241–4.

59. Mackenzie IR. The neuropathology and clinical phenotype of FTD with progranulin mutations. Acta Neuropathol 2007;114:49–54.

60. Baker M, Mackenzie IR, Pickering-Brown SM, et al. Mutations in progranulin cause tau-negative frontotemporal dementia linked to chromosome 17. Nature 2006;442:916–9.

61. Ahmed Z, Mackenzie IR, Hutton ML, et al. Progranulin in frontotemporal lobar degeneration and neuroinflammation. J Neuroinflammation 2007;4:7.

62. Goldman JS, Farmer JM, Van Deerlin VM, et al. Frontotemporal dementia: genetics and genetic counseling dilemmas. Neurologist 2004;10:227–34.

63. Geschwind D, Karrim J, Nelson SF, et al. The apolipoprotein E epsilon4 allele is not a significant risk factor for frontotemporal dementia. Ann Neurol 1998;44:134–8.

64. Agosta F, Vossel KA, Miller BL, et al. Apolipoprotein E epsilon4 is associated with disease-specific effects on brain atrophy in Alzheimer's disease and frontotemporal dementia. Proc Natl Acad Sci U S A 2009;106:2018–22.

65. Tartaglia MC, Laluz V, Rademakers R, et al. Polymorphism in Progranulin gene associated with structural differences in brains of normal controls. Neurology 2010;74.

66. Houlden H, Baker M, Morris HR, et al. Corticobasal degeneration and progressive supranuclear palsy share a common tau haplotype. Neurology 2001;56:1702–6.

67. Arai T, Hasegawa M, Akiyama H, et al. TDP-43 is a component of ubiquitin-positive tau-negative inclusions in frontotemporal lobar degeneration and amyotrophic lateral sclerosis. Biochem Biophys Res Commun 2006;351:602–11.

68. Rosen HJ, Gorno-Tempini ML, Goldman WP, et al. Patterns of brain atrophy in frontotemporal dementia and semantic dementia. Neurology 2002;58:198–208.

69. Whitwell JL, Josephs KA, Rossor MN, et al. Magnetic resonance imaging signatures of tissue pathology in frontotemporal dementia. Arch Neurol 2005;62:1402–8.

70. Rabinovici GD, Seeley WW, Kim EJ, et al. Distinct MRI atrophy patterns in autopsy-proven Alzheimer's disease and frontotemporal lobar degeneration. Am J Alzheimers Dis Other Demen 2007;22:474–88.

71. Seeley WW, Crawford RK, Zhou J, et al. Neurodegenerative diseases target large-scale human brain networks. Neuron 2009;62:42–52.

72. Kipps CM, Mioshi E, Hodges JR. Emotion, social functioning and activities of daily living in frontotemporal dementia. Neurocase 2009;15:182–9.

73. Phillips ML, Drevets WC, Rauch SL, et al. Neurobiology of emotion perception I: the neural basis of normal emotion perception. Biol Psychiatry 2003;54:504–14.

74. Rosen HJ, Allison SC, Ogar JM, et al. Behavioral features in semantic dementia vs other forms of progressive aphasias. Neurology 2006;67:1752–6.

75. Rosen HJ, Allison SC, Schauer GF, et al. Neuroanatomical correlates of behavioural disorders in dementia. Brain 2005;128:2612–25.

76. Rankin KP, Gorno-Tempini ML, Allison SC, et al. Structural anatomy of empathy in neurodegenerative disease. Brain 2006;129:2945–56.

77. Rankin KP, Salazar A, Gorno-Tempini ML, et al. Detecting sarcasm from paralinguistic cues: anatomic and cognitive correlates in neurodegenerative disease. Neuroimage 2009;47:2005–15.

78. Sollberger M, Stanley CM, Wilson SM, et al. Neural basis of interpersonal traits in neurodegenerative diseases. Neuropsychologia 2009;47:2812–27.

79. Rosen HJ, Wilson MR, Schauer GF, et al. Neuroanatomical correlates of impaired recognition of emotion in dementia. Neuropsychologia 2006;44:365–73.

80. Carey CL, Woods SP, Damon J, et al. Discriminant validity and neuroanatomical correlates of rule monitoring in frontotemporal dementia and Alzheimer's disease. Neuropsychologia 2008;46:1081–7.

81. Amici S, Brambati SM, Wilkins DP, et al. Anatomical correlates of sentence comprehension and verbal working memory in neurodegenerative disease. J Neurosci 2007;27:6282–90.

82. Wilson SM, Brambati SM, Henry RG, et al. The neural basis of surface dyslexia in semantic dementia. Brain 2009;132:71–86.

83. Rosen HJ, Alcantar O, Rothlind J, et al. Neuroanatomical correlates of cognitive self-appraisal in neurodegenerative disease. Neuroimage 2009;49:3358–64.

84. Thompson PM, Hayashi KM, de Zubicaray G, et al. Dynamics of gray matter loss in Alzheimer's disease. J Neurosci 2003;23:994–1005.

85. Seeley WW, Bauer AM, Miller BL, et al. The natural history of temporal variant frontotemporal dementia. Neurology 2005;64:1384–90.

86. Gorno-Tempini ML, Rankin KP, Woolley JD, et al. Cognitive and behavioral profile in a case of right anterior temporal lobe neurodegeneration. Cortex 2004;40:631–44.

87. Lee SE, Rabinovici GD, Mayo MC, et al. Clinicopathological correlations in corticobasal degeneration. Ann Neurol 2011;70:327–40.

88. Boxer AL, Geschwind MD, Belfor N, et al. Patterns of brain atrophy that differentiate corticobasal degeneration syndrome from progressive supranuclear palsy. Arch Neurol 2006;63:81–6.

89. Rohrer JD, Ridgway GR, Modat M, et al. Distinct profiles of brain atrophy in frontotemporal lobar degeneration caused by progranulin and tau mutations. Neuroimage 2010;53:1070–6.

90. Whitwell JL, Jack CR Jr, Boeve BF, et al. Voxel-based morphometry patterns of atrophy in FTLD with mutations in MAPT or PGRN. Neurology 2009;72:813–20.

91. Rohrer JD, Geser F, Zhou J, et al. TDP-43 subtypes are associated with distinct atrophy patterns in frontotemporal dementia. Neurology 2010;75:2204–11.

92. Neumann M, Kwong LK, Truax AC, et al. TDP-43-positive white matter pathology in frontotemporal lobar degeneration with ubiquitin-positive inclusions. J Neuropathol Exp Neurol 2007;66:177–83.

93. Zhukareva V, Mann D, Pickering-Brown S, et al. Sporadic Pick's disease: a tauopathy characterized by a spectrum of pathological tau isoforms in gray and white matter. Ann Neurol 2002;51:730–9.

94. Englund E. Neuropathology of white matter changes in Alzheimer's disease and vascular dementia. Dement Geriatr Cogn Disord 1998;9(Suppl 1):6–12.

95. Braak H, Braak E. Cortical and subcortical argyrophilic grains characterize a disease associated with adult onset dementia. Neuropathol Appl Neurobiol 1989;15:13–26.

96. Zhukareva V, Joyce S, Schuck T, et al. Unexpected abundance of pathological tau in progressive supranuclear palsy white matter. Ann Neurol 2006;60:335–45.

97. Dickson DW, Bergeron C, Chin SS, et al. Office of Rare Diseases neuropathologic criteria for corticobasal degeneration. J Neuropathol Exp Neurol 2002;61:935–46.

98. Chao LL, Schuff N, Clevenger EM, et al. Patterns of white matter atrophy in frontotemporal lobar degeneration. Arch Neurol 2007;64:1619–24.

99. Beaulieu C. The basis of anisotropic water diffusion in the nervous system–a technical review. NMR Biomed 2002;15:435–55.

100. Song SK, Sun SW, Ramsbottom MJ, et al. Dysmyelination revealed through MRI as increased radial (but unchanged axial) diffusion of water. Neuroimage 2002;17:1429–36.

101. Basser PJ, Mattiello J, LeBihan D. MR diffusion tensor spectroscopy and imaging. Biophys J 1994;66:259–67.

102. Zhang Y, Schuff N, Du AT, et al. White matter damage in frontotemporal dementia and Alzheimer's disease measured by diffusion MRI. Brain 2009;132:2579–92.

103. Galantucci S, Tartaglia MC, Wilson SM, et al. White matter damage in primary progressive aphasias: a diffusion tensor tractography study. Brain 2011;134(Pt 10):3011–29.

104. Gorno-Tempini ML, Brambati SM, Ginex V, et al. The logopenic/phonological variant of primary progressive aphasia. Neurology 2008;71:1227–34.

105. Tartaglia MC, Zhang Y, Racine C, et al. Executive dysfunction in frontotemporal dementia is related to abnormalities in frontal white matter tracts. Neurology 2009;72:A437.

106. Wilson SM, Galantucci S, Tartaglia MC, et al. Syntactic processing depends on dorsal language tracts. 2011;72(2):397–403.

107. Tartaglia MC, Galantucci S, Wilson SM, et al. White matter tract integrity corresponds with individual differences in emotional expression and sensitivity. Dement Geriatr Cognit Disord 2010;30(Suppl 1):84.

108. Fox MD, Corbetta M, Snyder AZ, et al. Spontaneous neuronal activity distinguishes human dorsal and ventral attention systems. Proc Natl Acad Sci U S A 2006;103:10046–51.

109. Seeley WW, Menon V, Schatzberg AF, et al. Dissociable intrinsic connectivity networks for salience processing and executive control. J Neurosci 2007;27:2349–56.

110. Smith SM, Fox PT, Miller KL, et al. Correspondence of the brain's functional architecture during activation and rest. Proc Natl Acad Sci U S A 2009;106:13040–5.

111. Fox MD, Snyder AZ, Vincent JL, et al. The human brain is intrinsically organized into dynamic, anti-correlated functional networks. Proc Natl Acad Sci U S A 2005;102:9673–8.

112. Greicius MD, Supekar K, Menon V, et al. Resting-state functional connectivity reflects structural connectivity in the default mode network. Cereb Cortex 2009;19:72–8.

113. Roberts DA, Detre JA, Bolinger L, et al. Quantitative magnetic resonance imaging of human brain perfusion at 1.5 T using steady-state inversion of arterial water. Proc Natl Acad Sci U S A 1994;91: 33–7.

114. Shimizu S, Zhang Y, Laxamana J, et al. Concordance and discordance between brain perfusion and atrophy in frontotemporal dementia. Brain Imaging Behav 2010;4:46–54.

115. Rabinovici GD, Furst AJ, O'Neil JP, et al. 11C-PIB PET imaging in Alzheimer disease and frontotemporal lobar degeneration. Neurology 2007;68:1205–12.

Reserve, Brain Changes, and Decline

Roger T. Staff, PhD

KEYWORDS

- Brain reserve • Reserve models • Brain genetics
- Dementia

Reserve is a heuristic concept used to explain the apparent discrepancy between pathologic changes in the brain normally associated with aging and disease, and the manifestation of those changes in terms of clinical presentation and cognitive decline. It has been used to explain this discrepancy in a range of situations such as multiple sclerosis,[1] dementia,[2] and individual differences in cognitive aging.[3] It is not the intention of this article to document an anthology of research concerned directly or indirectly with reserve, but to provide an overview of the concepts and applications being used to explore reserve and proposed connections between empiric proxies of reserve, hypothesized biological mechanisms, and the protection from aging and disease that reserve imparts.

A BRIEF HISTORY OF RESERVE

Interest in reserve has steadily increased since the early 1990s, with a Web of Science search identifying 138 publications using the term (or similar) in 2010 and more than 1200 publications since 1990. One of most frequently cited publications that refers to reserve is by Katzman and colleagues[4] in 1988, who noted that those individuals with high levels of Alzheimer's disease (AD) pathology post mortem, who otherwise remained nondemented in life, had almost double the number of large pyramidal neurons throughout their neocortex in comparison with those who expressed clinical symptoms. This publication goes on to suggest that those nondemented in life might have started with a larger brain and more neurons and thus might be said to possess greater reserve against incipient AD, but did not become clinically demented because of this greater reserve.

Although this is a modern articulation, the concept of brain reserve is not new. In the 1960s work done in and around Newcastle upon Tyne in the United Kingdom noted "it would appear that a certain amount of the change estimated by plaque counts may be accommodated within the reserve capacity of the cerebrum without causing manifest intellectual impairment,"[5] and that "although the association between dementia and brain degeneration is impressive the extent of the degeneration varies considerably; moreover, occasionally, the brains of individuals who have never become demented have been found to show quite marked changes." Moreover, "the condition of the brain seems therefore to be only one of several factors determining the threshold at which dementia appears."[6] Collectively these publications make two clear points: (1) the brain has a buffer or reserve capacity to withstand a degree of change brought about by aging and disease, and (2) the size of that capacity is different between individuals.

Although less scientifically vigorous, publications from the early twentieth century discuss the concept of reserve in mediating behavior in the face of pathologic change. Pickworth[7] in the 1930s comments that "no clinical abnormality is noticed unless the damage is quantitatively so great as to exceed the reserve." Indeed, Flemming[8] in the 1920s goes as far as to suggest how reserve is acquired. "...The great storehouse for personal memories, the residue of individual experience. These reserves are drawn on to cooperate in deciding, on the basis of personal as well as racial experience, what act is appropriate to the situation." These early publications are by no means the only two to articulate the concept of reserve in the early twentieth century.

Aberdeen Royal Infirmary, Department of Bio-Medical Physics, NHS-Grampian and the University of Aberdeen, Foresterhill, Aberdeen AB25 2ZD, Scotland, UK
E-mail address: r.staff@abdn.ac.uk

Neuroimag Clin N Am 22 (2012) 99–105
doi:10.1016/j.nic.2011.11.006

neuroimaging.theclinics.com

With the increased availability of modern imaging techniques, the discrepancy between brain changes characteristic of disease and aging and an individual's clinical presentation or cognitive performance has been reemphasized. The advent of specific β-amyloid (Aβ) ligands for positron emission tomography (PET), such as Pittsburgh compound B (PIB), has brought about great optimism for a new era in AD imaging diagnosis. However, not all patients with positive PIB PET have or develop AD.[9] This fact may be attributable to the lack of specificity of the ligand and/or the exact role of Aβ in the development of AD, but it is also consistent with the notion that individual differences in reserve allow some people to maintain function in the face of disease-like pathologic burden. Similarly, a study using ^{18}F-fluorodeoxyglucose (FDG) PET indicated that some individuals (those with more years of schooling) were able to maintain function in the face of similar metabolic deficits.[10] Stern and colleagues[11] found that AD patients with more education had larger regional cerebral blood flow (rCBF) deficits, measured using single-photon emission computed tomography (SPECT), suggesting that more education enabled an individual to cope with greater levels of pathologic change. Reed and colleagues[2] showed that schooling attenuates the cognitive effect of brain atrophy measured using magnetic resonance (MR) imaging.

RESERVE MODELS

It is unclear how reserve enables an individual to withstand the effects of age and disease-related pathologic change. Stern[12] has suggested conceptual models for reserve and postulates different mechanisms for the implementation of reserve; the first he refers to as "brain reserve," suggesting that individuals have different amounts of brain reserve and that, for a given amount of pathologic burden, those with more reserve will be less affected. This brain reserve could, therefore, be said to passively protect an individual against the effect aging and disease. Structural proxies of passive brain reserve suggested in the literature are indices such as brain or head volume,[13] head circumference,[14] synaptic count,[15] or dendritic branching.[16]

An active mechanism through which function is maintained has also been proposed, which has been described as cognitive reserve. An individual with this type of reserve uses brain networks or cognitive paradigms that are less susceptible to disruption and could be said to have "neural reserve."[17] The second mechanism is described as neural compensation. Here, in the face of

pathology, the brain recruits structures and/or networks not normally used by individuals with intact brains, to compensate for pathologic burden. The literature has consistently identified proxies of active or cognitive reserve, such as premorbid cognitive ability, education, physical activity, intellectual engagement, and occupational attainment. These insightful models have structured reserve research and have provided a vocabulary with which to discuss the phenomenon.

These models may not be as discrete as they first appear and are not mutually exclusive. When examining brain reserve proxies, it is clear from the literature that these measures have also been shown to be modifiable through intervention and the environment. For example, McEwen[18] has suggested that repeated stressors result in decreased dendritic branching and a reduction in the number of neurons. It has recently been suggested that early-life experience has a significant association with late-life brain size[19] and may also be considered as a lifelong proxy of cognitive reserve. Therefore, brain reserve may represent, at least in part, the integration of life experience and environmental factors that overlap with the proxies of cognitive reserve. For example, a common proxy for cognitive reserve is education.[20] Education is not only associated with premorbid ability but is influenced by childhood socioeconomic status,[19] which in turn may reflect individual differences in diet and early-life stimulation. Moreover, education may influence late-life socioeconomic status and intellectual engagement, which may have an impact through passive and/or active routes. These structural, probably causal, paths between potential measures of reserve that extend across all models would suggest that reserve is unlikely to be optimally described by a single factor that can be measured directly.

Brain Reserve and the Passive Model

The passive reserve model can be summarized by the phrase "the more you have the more you have to lose before deficits appear." "Having more" brain reserve, such as more synapses, will lead to sufficient residual capacity after accounting for pathology for function to continue unaltered. Insufficient reserve will lead to inadequate capacity, and functional loss will occur. There is considerable observational evidence that is consistent with the passive reserve model. Studies[4,21,22] have reported higher levels of reserve proxies, such as brain size, neuronal number, and neuronal density in individuals with brain changes associated with dementia and disease but little or no cognitive deficits.

Cognitive Reserve and the Active Model

The active reserve model proposes that individual differences in processing mechanisms and the ability to compensate by actively adapting these mechanisms (and using new ones) is responsible for protecting an individual against the detrimental cognitive effects of aging and disease. A person's premorbid intelligence as well as educational and occupational attainment have been suggested as proxies for measuring this ability. These measures are assumed to reflect the neural efficiency, or the ability to recruit alternative brain networks to compensate, when faced with pathology. Epidemiologic evidence supports the active or cognitive reserve hypothesis, with lower baseline intelligence scores, less education, and lower occupational attainment being risk factors for dementia and cognitive decline.[23,24]

A processing mechanism that is less susceptible to pathology is a potential source of cognitive reserve. Consider two individuals who perform identically through different neuronal routes because they have different brain structures or different expertise and training, or who might have used different cognitive strategies. One may be considered to have reserve if the mechanisms used are less susceptible to aging and disease. Evidence for individual differences such as these has been considered in a review article by Deary and colleagues.[25] An alternative source of active reserve has its origins in an individual's ability to compensate for detrimental pathology. This reserve could be realized by upregulation of an existing mechanism (working harder) or by the recruitment of alternative or more extensive neural networks (doing different). A recent review by Eyler and colleagues[26] into the functional brain imaging correlates of successful cognitive aging reported "frequent support for the notion that increased brain responsiveness is associated with better cognitive performance" in aging samples. However, it is unclear whether this increased responsiveness is a consequence of the better performers' mechanisms of working harder or doing different. or whether better performers had increased responsiveness before the onset of pathologic burden and established mechanisms that are less susceptible to disease and aging. Or is it the case that a combination of all possible sources and mechanisms of reserve is required to cope with the onset of disease and aging? It is difficult to test for the presence of one strategy versus another using a cross-sectional, observational approach predominantly used in the field. For example; Persson and colleagues[27] compared the frontal cortex functional (fMR) imaging response during a verbal encoding task between those who had stable memory performance and those who had declined. Greater response was found in the right ventral prefrontal cortex among decliners than in those with stable performance. Is this evidence of a declining person working harder or are those that develop more efficient mechanisms being less susceptible? Cabeza and colleagues[28] found that young adults and poorer performing older adults recruited similar right prefrontal cortex (PFC) regions, whereas higher performing older adults engaged PFC regions bilaterally. The investigators concluded that poorer performing older adults recruit a network of brain regions similar to those of young adults, but use these inefficiently, whereas higher performing older adults compensate for age-related neural decline by reorganizing brain functions, that is to say, doing different in that face of aging. An alternative explanation would be that higher performing adults develop this alternative mechanism before the onset of aging pathology and are therefore less susceptible.

ACQUIRING RESERVE GENETICALLY

There is of course no randomized, double-blind longitudinal intervention study to identify the elements or life experiences that contribute to reserve. Evidence that reserve can be acquired is observational in nature, and causality is inferred rather than proved. It may well be that the proxies attributed to reserve are not causal but correlative and have, at least in part, a common origin. Examining the acquisition of brain or cognitive reserve separately is difficult because the parameters that describe a life course are interconnected. A genetically endowed advantage leading to greater neuronal numbers and a larger brain will also influence early-life intelligence, the education one receives, one's occupational attainment, and the intellectual and physical pursuits one chooses to undertake. The influence of this life-course description of reserve is further complicated by the potential of the avoidance of pathologic burden by the educated and/or affluent. That is, those in privileged positions may avoid the potential risk factors for dementia, such as toxic exposures and risks encountered by manual workers, and are better able to act on public health advice by taking regular exercise and not smoking.

Genetic and environmental factors will influence an individual's response to aging and disease. The combination of genes and environmental factors influencing brain development may also influence reserve and may be just as important, either alone or in combination, in early life as they are later. Identifying the genetic risk factors for dementia is a rapidly growing field, with most (but not all) candidate genes having a likely hypothesized mechanism from genotype, through pathology, to disease.[29]

Identifying the genetic contributions to reserve holistically is difficult because of the absence of a directly measurable reserve quantity. There is considerable evidence that heritability is responsible for brain (and thus head) size, measures considered as proxies of passive brain reserve. Bartley and colleagues,[30] examining twins using structural MR imaging, concluded that human cerebral size is determined almost entirely by genetic factors, but that overall cortical gyral pattern, though significantly influenced by genes, is determined primarily by nongenetic factors. Pfefferbaum and colleagues,[31] examining twins in the seventh and eighth decades of life, found that both genetic and environmental influences contribute to the variability of brain structure, but that the manner in which the brain responds to the environment with advancing age is highly genetically determined.

Similarly there is considerable evidence for a genetic influence on measures of premorbid cognitive ability, which has been considered as a proxy of reserve. Family and twins studies support genetic contributions to cognitive ability and reserve.[32] Heritability explains a significant proportion of the normal variation in human cognition, with the proportion depending on how cognition was tested. Swan and Carmelli[33] found executive function to be highly heritable. Executive function has also been shown to decline with age.[34] Taken together, these findings suggest that cognitive ability and subsequently the rate of age-related cognitive decline are highly heritable. There are reliable associations in older people between apolipoprotein E (APOE) polymorphisms and dementia, with multiple pathways that may explain the pathogenic nature of APOE.[35] These factors include its role in the formation of AD neuropathology but also its role in modifying synaptic plasticity and repair. Reduced plasticity may well influence age-related neural reorganizing of brain functions, a postulated compensatory mechanism of reserve (doing different).

The genetic influence of brain connectivity has recently been examined by Fornito and colleagues,[36] who used fMR imaging to study twins and identified genetic influences on anatomic connectivity. Extrapolating from this work, it is reasonable to suggest that different levels of connectivity may facilitate more robust and/or different mechanisms that maintain cognition in the face of pathologic burden. Examining the influence of APOE genotype, Dennis and colleagues[37] found that in the absence of demographic or performance differences, carriers of APOE epsilon 4 (ε4) allele exhibited greater bilateral medial temporal lobe activity relative to noncarriers (working harder) while accomplishing the same encoding task. In addition, APOE ε4 carriers demonstrated a greater functional connectivity to some regions, but overall reductions in connectivity were found across the anterior and posterior cortices. Brain regions implicated in this investigation are known to incur structural and functional changes in mild cognitive impairment and AD. The investigators attribute these differences in connectivity patterns to the APOE-driven pleiotropism in functional brain organization in early life. These individual differences may enable mechanisms that are less susceptible to aging and disease burden, or may facilitate compensatory mechanisms (doing different) in the face of pathologic burden.

ACQUIRING RESERVE ENVIRONMENTALLY

Without considering genetic predisposition, risk factors for cognitive decline and dementia are interrelated, and probably have an impact on both the accumulation of dementia-related neuropathological burden and the acquisition of reserve. Experiences during life that are considered to promote reserve are socioeconomic status,[38] social engagement,[39] education, occupational status,[3] mental engagement, and physical activity.[40]

A complete model for the interconnectivity and structure has yet to be established but, using a life-course approach, childhood socioeconomic status has been shown to influence childhood cognitive ability, education, occupational attainment, and cognition in late middle age in a variety of direct and indirect causal pathways.[41] Similarly, Hirvensalo and Lintunen[42] have suggested that socioeconomic status influences physical activity and, subsequently, health. Social engagement is related to cognition throughout adulthood, and is an important factor to consider in relation to efforts to promote optimal cognitive development and cognitive aging.[43]

Although there is empirical evidence for these proxies of reserve, the biological mechanisms through which these environmental factors act to realize reserve are unclear. Staff and colleagues[19] recently demonstrated an association between socioeconomic position in childhood and hippocampal volumes in late life, and suggested that childhood socioeconomic status brings about other individual differences, for example in education, occupation, diet, and mental stimulation, which result in restricted development of the hippocampus. Hippocampal volume is a risk factor for conversion to AD.[44] Hippocampal volume may then be considered a proxy of passive reserve (having more). Similarly, Rushton and Ankney[45] showed in a cross-sectional study that brain size increased with socioeconomic status. This mechanism of passive reserve may explain the association between risk of dementia and socioeconomic position.

Alternatively, these proxies of passive reserve may bring about mechanisms and connectivity patterns that facilitate active mechanisms. This proposal is partly conjecture, but Corden and colleagues[46] found that those with high social cognition scores activated a different network when compared with those with lower social cognition scores. Social cognition has been shown to be associated with social interaction/engagement.[47] The causal direction is unproven; however, the reserve provided by greater social engagement may be a consequence of the use of different neuronal networks, with the high social cognition network being less susceptible to burden. Song and colleagues[48] found that functional connectivity within the frontal lobe and between the frontal and posterior brain regions were both important predictive factors for intelligence. This connectivity may well facilitate the formation of less susceptible mechanisms through greater efficiency, or provide an individual with more compensatory options in the face of burden (doing different).

Waiter and colleagues,[49] using fMR imaging response to the inspection time task in two groups aged 69 years who differed in terms of their lifelong cognitive trajectory, found that the group of individuals who maintained their cognitive ability, relative to their childhood ability, demonstrated a pattern similar to healthy young samples. It is reasonable to assume that maintenance of cognitive ability was brought about by factors such education, occupation, and intellectual engagement, resulting in the network responsible for the task being less susceptible. In addition, the different pattern observed in those that had a less favorable lifelong cognitive trajectory may be evidence of a functional relocation of the network responsible for the task (doing different) in those experiencing preclinical cognitive decline, or possibly evidence that those with less intellectual enrichment throughout life had always relied on a different neuronal network that was more susceptible to decline.

TESTING AND MEASURING RESERVE

This article hypothesizes the potential links between proxies of reserve, differences in brain structure, functional architecture, adaptability, and the protection from functional loss. To test the reserve hypothesis requires a proxy estimate of reserve, a measure of pathologic burden in the brain, and a measure of cognitive change. This evaluation can only be accurately achieved using imaging in a longitudinal study design for a well-characterized sample. Although cross-sectional investigations still have a role to play in linking reserve proxies to brain differences and brain differences to cognitive change, the subtle interrelationships of reserve will best be exposed with long-term longitudinal studies.

Bolstering reserve is an obvious therapeutic target with which to counteract the effects of brain aging and dementia. The field, however, is limited by the use of proxy or surrogate measures for reserve, such as the participation in complex mental activities (education, occupation, social engagement) or crude biological markers (head size, brain volumes). The evolving imaging fields that measure anatomic and functional connectivity[36] and the use of information/systems theory approaches to examine qualities such as robustness[50] may provide more insightful biological measures of reserve. A true measure of reserve should explain a large proportion of the remaining variance in cognition, after adjusting for the influence of neuropathologic burden. The more variance it explains, the better the measure. A secondary feature should be that the environmental or biological proxy of reserve has biologically plausible mechanisms of action. Creating a practical measure that successfully aggregates the possible sources of reserve would enable identification of vulnerable groups for intervention, and enable researchers to better predict decline and subsequently quantify the influence of any intervention.

SUMMARY

Current evidence indicates that there are many roads to reserve, all of which are interconnected. It is likely that these have their origins in early life through genetic predisposition, but are modifiable throughout life. Simplifying the categories of having more, being more or less susceptible, working harder, and doing different have been used for convenience, and do not imply that they are discrete; indeed, having more neurons is likely to facilitate more than one mechanism of reserve. Despite the considerable literature on the subject, reserve remains a heuristic concept with only portions of the full picture currently understood.

REFERENCES

1. Benedict RH, Morrow SA, Guttman BW, et al. Cognitive reserve moderates decline in information

processing speed in multiple sclerosis patients. J Int Neuropsychol Soc 2010;16:829–35.

2. Reed BR, Mungas D, Farias ST, et al. Measuring cognitive reserve based on the decomposition of episodic memory variance RID E-6810-2011 RID B-5541-2009. Brain 2010;133:2196–209.

3. Staff R, Murray A, Deary I, et al. What provides cerebral reserve? RID C-6297-2009 RID E-9019-2011. Brain 2004;127:1191–9.

4. Katzman R, Terry R, Deteresa R, et al. Clinical, pathological, and neurochemical changes in dementia—a subgroup with preserved mental status and numerous neocortical plaques. Ann Neurol 1988; 23:138–44.

5. Blessed G, Tomlinson BE, Roth M. The association between quantitative measures of dementia and of senile change in the grey matter of elderly subjects. Br J Psychiatry 1967;114:797.

6. Kay DW, Beamish P, Roth M. Old age mental disorders in Newcastle upon Tyne. Br J Psychiatry 1964;110:146.

7. Pickworth FA. The pathology of the nasal sinuses and its relation to mental disorder. J Ment Sci 1932;78:635.

8. Fleming GW. A further contribution to the psychology of the essential epileptic. J Ment Sci 1927;73:141.

9. Rabinovici GD, Jagust WJ. Amyloid imaging in aging and dementia: testing the amyloid hypothesis in vivo. Behav Neurol 2009;21:117–28.

10. Perneczky R, Drzezga A, Diehl-Schmid J, et al. Schooling mediates brain reserve in Alzheimer's disease: findings of fluoro-deoxy-glucose positron emission tomography. J Neurol Neurosurg Psychiatry 2006;77:1060–3.

11. Stern Y, Alexander G, Prohovnik I, et al. Inverse relationship between education and parietotemporal perfusion deficit in Alzheimers disease. Ann Neurol 1992;32:371–5.

12. Stern Y. What is cognitive reserve? Theory and research application of the reserve concept. J Int Neuropsychol Soc 2002;8:448–60.

13. Mortimer JA, Borenstein AR, Gosche KM, et al. Very early detection of Alzheimer neuropathology and the role of brain reserve in modifying its clinical expression. J Geriatr Psychiatry Neurol 2005;18:218–23.

14. Perneczky R, Wagenpfeil S, Lunetta KL, et al. Head circumference, atrophy, and cognition. Neurology 2010;75:137–42.

15. Petrosini L, De Bartolo P, Foti F, et al. On whether the environmental enrichment may provide cognitive and brain reserves RID D-1269-2010. Brain Res Rev 2009;61:221–39.

16. Vance DE, Roberson AJ, McGuinness TM, et al. How neuroplasticity and cognitive reserve protect cognitive functioning. J Psychosoc Nurs Ment Health Serv 2010;48:23–30.

17. Stern Y. Cognitive reserve and Alzheimer disease. Alzheimer Dis Assoc Disord 2006;20:112–7.

18. McEwen BS. Protective and damaging effects of stress mediators. N Engl J Med 1998;338:171–9.

19. Staff RT, Murray AD, Ahearn TS, et al. Childhood socioeconomic status and adult brain size. Ann Neurol, in press.

20. Murray AD, Staff RT, McNeil CJ, et al. The balance between cognitive reserve and brain imaging biomarkers of cerebrovascular and Alzheimer's diseases. Brain, in press.

21. Mortimer J. Brain reserve and the clinical expression of Alzheimer's disease. Geriatrics 1997;52: S50–3.

22. den Heijer T, Geerlings M, Hoebeek F, et al. Use of hippocampal and amygdalar volumes on magnetic resonance imaging to predict dementia in cognitively intact elderly people. Arch Gen Psychiatry 2006;63:57–62.

23. Katzman R. Education and the prevalence of dementia and Alzheimers disease. Neurology 1993;43:13–20.

24. Letenneur L, Gilleron V, Commenges D, et al. Are sex and educational level independent predictors of dementia and Alzheimer's disease? Incidence data from the PAQUID project. J Neurol Neurosurg Psychiatry 1999;66:177–83.

25. Deary IJ, Penke L, Johnson W. The neuroscience of human intelligence differences RID C-6297-2009. Nat Rev Neurosci 2010;11:201–11.

26. Eyler LT, Sherzai A, Kaup AR, et al. A review of functional brain imaging correlates of successful cognitive aging. Biol Psychiatry 2011;70:115–22.

27. Persson J, Nyberg L, Lind J, et al. Structure-function correlates of cognitive decline in aging RID C-2514-2009. Cereb Cortex 2006;16:907–15.

28. Cabeza R, Anderson N, Locantore J, et al. Aging gracefully: compensatory brain activity in high-performing older adults RID E-9101-2011. Neuroimage 2002;17:1394–402.

29. Serretti A, Olgiati P, De Ronchi D. Genetics of Alzheimer's disease. A rapidly evolving field. J Alzheimers Dis 2007;12:73–92.

30. Bartley A, Jones D, Weinberger D. Genetic variability of human brain size and cortical gyral patterns. Brain 1997;120:257–69.

31. Pfefferbaum A, Sullivan E, Swan G, et al. Brain structure in men remains highly heritable in the seventh and eighth decades of life. Neurobiol Aging 2000; 21:63–74.

32. Lee J. Genetic evidence for cognitive reserve: variations in memory and related cognitive functions. J Clin Exp Neuropsychol 2003;25:594–613.

33. Swan G, Carmelli D. Evidence for genetic mediation of executive control: a study of aging male twins. J Gerontol B Psychol Sci Soc Sci 2002;57: P133–43.

34. McPherson S, Fairbanks L, Tiken S, et al. Apathy and executive function in Alzheimer's disease. J Int Neuropsychol Soc 2002;8:373–81.

35. Bu G. Apolipoprotein E and its receptors in Alzheimer's disease: pathways, pathogenesis and therapy. Nat Rev Neurosci 2009;10:333–44.

36. Fornito A, Zalesky A, Bassett DS, et al. Genetic influences on cost-efficient organization of human cortical functional networks RID F-2466-2011. J Neurosci 2011;31:3261–70.

37. Dennis NA, Browndyke JN, Stokes J, et al. Temporal lobe functional activity and connectivity in young adult APOE epsilon 4 carriers. Alzheimers Dement 2010;6:303–11.

38. Glymour MM, Manly JJ. Lifecourse social conditions and racial and ethnic patterns of cognitive aging. Neuropsychol Rev 2008;18:223–54.

39. Wang H, Karp A, Winblad B, et al. Late-life engagement in social and leisure activities is associated with a decreased risk of dementia: a longitudinal study from the Kungsholmen project. Am J Epidemiol 2002;155:1081–7.

40. Fratiglioni L, Paillard-Borg S, Winblad B. An active and socially integrated lifestyle in late life might protect against dementia. Lancet Neurol 2004;3: 343–53.

41. Richards M, Sacker A. Lifetime antecedents of cognitive reserve. J Clin Exp Neuropsychol 2003; 25:614–24.

42. Hirvensalo M, Lintunen T. Life-course perspective for physical activity and sports participation. Eur Rev Aging Phys Act 2011;8:13–22.

43. Seeman TE, Miller-Martinez DM, Merkin SS, et al. Histories of social engagement and adult cognition: midlife in the U.S. study. J Gerontol B Psychol Sci Soc Sci 2011;66:141–52.

44. Jack C, Petersen R, Xu Y, et al. Prediction of AD with MRI-based hippocampal volume in mild cognitive impairment RID F-2508-2010. Neurology 1999;52: 1397–403.

45. Rushton J, Ankney C. Brain size and cognitive ability: correlations with age, sex, social class, and race. Psychon Bull Rev 1996;3:21–36.

46. Corden B, Critchley HD, Skuse D, et al. Fear recognition ability predicts differences in social cognitive and neural functioning in men. J Cogn Neurosci 2006;18:889–97.

47. Amodio DM, Frith CD. Meeting of minds: the medial frontal cortex and social cognition. Nature 2006;7: 268.

48. Song M, Zhou Y, Li J, et al. Brain spontaneous functional connectivity and intelligence RID F-2682-2011. Neuroimage 2008;41:1168–76.

49. Waiter GD, Fox HC, Murray AD, et al. Is retaining the youthful functional anatomy underlying speed of information processing a signature of successful cognitive ageing? An event-related fMRI study of inspection time performance RID C-8951-2011 RID E-9019-2011 RID C-6297-2009. Neuroimage 2008; 41:581–95.

50. Sokumbi MO, Staff RT, Waiter GD, et al. Inter-individual differences in fMRI entropy measurements in old age. IEEE Trans Biomed Eng 2011;58(11): 3206–14.

The Clinical Value of Large Neuroimaging Data Sets in Alzheimer's Disease

Arthur W. Toga, PhD

KEYWORDS

- Neuroimaging • Database • Alzheimer's disease
- Informatics

Rapid advances over the past several decades in neuroimaging and cyberinfrastructure technologies have brought explosive growth in the Web-based warehousing, availability, and accessibility of imaging data on a broad array of neurodegenerative and neuropsychiatric disorders and conditions.[1–4] This growth has been driven largely by the demand for multiscale data in the investigation of fundamental disease processes; the need for interdisciplinary cooperation to integrate, question, and interpret the data; and the movement of science in general toward freely available and openly accessible information. In response to this substantial need for capacity to store and exchange data online in meaningful ways in support of data analysis, hypothesis testing, and future reanalysis or even repurposing, the electronic collection, organization, annotation, storage, and distribution of clinical, genetic, and imaging data are essential activities in the contemporary biomedical and translational discovery process. The result has been the prolific development and emergence of complex computational infrastructures that serve as repositories of databases and provide critical functionalities such as sophisticated image analysis algorithm pipelines and powerful three-dimensional (3D) visualization and statistical tools.[5–9] The statistical and operational advantages of collaborative, distributed team science in the form of multisite consortia continue to push this approach in a diverse range of population-based investigations.

NEW ERA OF COLLABORATIVE, INTERDISCIPLINARY TEAM SCIENCE

The ongoing convergence and integration of neuroscientific infrastructures worldwide is heading to the creation of a global virtual imaging laboratory. Through ordinary Web browsers, large-scale image data sets and related clinical data and biospecimens, algorithm pipelines, computational resources, and visualization and statistical toolkits are easily accessible to users regardless of their physical location or disciplinary orientation. The promise of this investigatory environment-without-walls, and its incipient marshalling of scientific talent and facilitation of collaboration across multiple disciplines, are accelerating various translational initiatives with high societal impact, such as early or presymptomatic diagnosis and prevention of Alzheimer's disease (AD).

Neuroimaging is now a major focus for multi-institutional research on progressive changes in brain architecture, biomarkers of treatment response, and the differential effects of disease on patterns of cognitive activation and connectivity.[10] Prominent research consortia and multisite clinical trials have focused on AD, pediatric brain cancer, and fetal alcohol syndrome, in addition to multi-institutional collaborative programs for mapping the normal brain.[11,12] Current leading-edge mapping consortia are focusing on the human brain as a complex network of connectivity and aim for a comprehensive structural description of the network architecture of the brain.[13] This

Laboratory of Neuro Imaging, Department of Neurology, David Geffen School of Medicine at UCLA, 635 Charles Young Drive S, Suite 225, Los Angeles, CA 90095-7334, USA
E-mail address: toga@loni.ucla.edu

Neuroimag Clin N Am 22 (2012) 107–118
doi:10.1016/j.nic.2011.11.008
1052-5149/12/$ – see front matter © 2012 Elsevier Inc. All rights reserved.

collaborative effort, the human connectome (http://www.humanconnectomeproject.org/), is exploring and generating new insights in to the organization of the structural connections of the brain and their role in shaping functional dynamics and brain plasticity. Such large-scale efforts necessitate close coordination of image data collection protocols, ontology development, computational requirements, and sharing.

IMPACT OF KEY AREAS OF E-SCIENCE ON NEUROSCIENCE AND NEUROLOGY

Multisite neuroimaging studies are dramatically accelerating the pace and volume of discoveries regarding major brain disease and the contrasts between normal and abnormal brain structure and function.[14] The large-scale, purpose-driven data sets generated by these consortia can then be used by the broader community to model and predict clinical outcomes as well as guide clinicians in selecting treatment options for various neurologic diseases. Multisite trials are an important element in the study of a disease or the process of evaluating an intervention. Linking together multiple sites facilitates the recruitment of large samples that yield high statistical power for both main analyses as well as secondary analyses of subgroups. Generalizability of results to the level of the population is also maximized. Because data come from multiple sites, investigators can explore how the effects of a treatment vary across geographically diverse sites and how such variation relates to site characteristics, and to cultural and socioeconomic characteristics of the patients who participated in the studies. Such information can directly inform clinical decision-making at the level of the patient and guide the selection of treatment options. These research efforts are imperative for guiding treatment recommendations for neurologic disorders domestically and internationally as well as at the level of the individual patient. Multicenter collaborations strengthen understanding of brain diseases that affect all walks of life, all ages, and all cultures, thus enabling accelerated translation of neuroimaging trial outcomes directly into clinical applications.

Large archives of neuroimaging data are also creating innumerable opportunities for reanalysis and mining that can lead to new findings of use in basic research or in the characterization of clinical syndromes. Access to databases of neuroanatomic morphology has led to the development of content-driven approaches for exploration of brains that are anatomically similar, revealing patterns embedded within entire (sub)sets of neuroimaging data.[4]

Provenance, or the description of the history of a set of data, has grown more important with the proliferation of research consortia-related efforts in neuroimaging.[5,12,15] Knowledge about the origin and history of an image is crucial for establishing the quality of data and results; detailed information about how it was processed, including the specific software routines and operating systems that were used, is necessary for proper interpretation, high-fidelity replication, and reuse and repurposing of the data. New mechanisms have emerged for describing provenance in a simple and easy-to-use environment, alleviating the burden of documentation from the user and still providing a rich description of the source history of an image. This combination of ease of use and highly descriptive metadata is greatly facilitating the collection of provenance and subsequent sharing of large data sets.

Multimodal classification of images has advanced the usefulness of atlases of neuropathology through standardized 3D coordinate systems that integrate data across patients, techniques, and acquisitions.[11,16,17] Atlases with a well-defined coordinate space, together with algorithms to align data with them, have enabled the pooling of brain mapping data from multiple subjects and sources, including large patient populations, and facilitated reconstruction of the trajectories of neurodegenerative diseases like AD as they progress in the living brain.[18–22] Automated algorithms can then use atlas descriptions of anatomic variance to guide image segmentation, tissue classification, functional analysis, and detection of disease.[7,23,24] Statistical representations of anatomy resulting from the application of atlasing strategies to specific subgroups of diseased individuals have revealed characteristics of structural brain differences in many diseases, including AD, human immunodeficiency virus/AIDS, unipolar depression, Tourette syndrome, and autism.[25]

Atlas-based descriptions of variance offer statistics on degenerative rates and can elucidate clinically relevant features at the systems level. Atlases have identified differences in atrophic patterns between AD and Lewy body dementia, and differences between atrophy rates across clinically defined subtypes of psychosis. Atlases have also revealed the association between genes and brain structure.[26] Based on well-characterized patient groups, population-based atlases contain composite maps and visualizations of structural variability, asymmetry, and group-specific differences. Pathologic change can be tracked over time, and generic features resolved, enabling these atlases to offer biomarkers for a variety of pathologic conditions as well as morphometric measures for genetic studies or drug trials.

Brain atlases can now accommodate observations from multiple modalities and from populations of individuals collected at different laboratories around the world. These probabilistic systems show promise for identifying patterns of structural, functional, and molecular variation in large imaging databases, for disease detection in individuals and groups, and for determining the effects of age, gender, handedness, and other demographic or genetic factors on brain structures in space and time. Integrating these observations to enable statistical comparison has already provided a deeper understanding of the relationship between brain structure and function.

This article considers and assesses the clinical implications of enabling large numbers of scientists to work in tandem with the same large data sets in the context of one such effort, the Alzheimer's Disease Neuroimaging Initiative (ADNI). Two facets, in particular, of this project exemplify the clinical value of large-scale neuroimaging databases in research and in patient care: (1) disease diagnosis and progression tracking, including the diagnostic value of image databases in demarcating abnormal and normal ranges of biospecimens; and (2) role of neuroimages in statistical powering, subject stratification, and incisive end points and outcomes of clinical trials.

ADNI

ADNI exemplifies a remarkably successful, open, shared, and efficient database.[27–30] ADNI brings together geographically distributed investigators with diverse scientific capabilities for the intensive study of biomarkers that signify and track the progression of AD. The quantity of imaging, clinical, cognitive, biochemical, and genetic data acquired and generated throughout the project have required powerful informatics systems and mechanisms for processing, integrating, and disseminating these data not only to support the research needs of the investigators who make up the ADNI cores but also to provide widespread data access to the greater scientific community. At the junction of this collaborative endeavor, the University of California at Los Angeles Laboratory of Neuro Imaging (LONI) has provided an infrastructure to facilitate data integration, access, and sharing across a diverse and growing community of multidisciplinary scientists.

ADNI is composed of 8 cores responsible for conducting the study along with external investigators authorized to use ADNI data. The various

information systems used by the cores result in an intricate flow of data in to, out of, and among information systems and institutions. The data flow into the ADNI data repository (http://adni.loni.ucla.edu/), where they are made available to the community. This well-curated scientific data repository enables data to be accessed by researchers across the globe and to be preserved over time. More than 1300 investigators have been granted access to ADNI data, resulting in extensive download activity that exceeds 1 million downloads of imaging, clinical, biomarker, and genetic data.

Image Data Workflow

The ADNI informatics core provides a user-friendly, Web-based environment for storing, searching, and sharing data acquired and generated by the ADNI community. In the process, the LONI image and data archive (IDA) has grown to meet the evolving needs of the ADNI community through continuing development of an increasingly interactive environment for data discovery and visualization. The automated systems developed to date include components for deidentification and secure archiving of imaging data from the 57 ADNI sites; management of the image workflow whereby raw images move from quarantine status to general availability and then proceed through preprocessing and postprocessing stages; integration of nonimaging data from other cores; management of data access and data sharing activities; and provision of a central, secure repository for disseminating data and related information to the ADNI community.

The imaging cores perform quality control and preprocessing of the magnetic resonance (MR) and positron emission tomography (PET) images; the ADNI image analysts perform postprocessing and analysis of the preprocessed images and related data; the biochemical samples are processed and the results compiled; and investigators download and analyze data as best fits their individual research needs.

Raw image data

In keeping with the objectives of the ADNI project to make data available to the scientific community, without embargo, and meet the needs of the core investigators, the IDA developed the image data workflow shown in **Fig. 1**. Initially, each acquisition site uploads image data to the repository via the IDA, a Web-based application that incorporates several data validation and data deidentification operations, including validation of the subject identifier, validation of the dataset as human or phantom, validation of the file format, image file

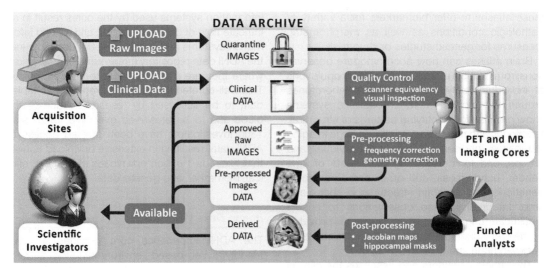

Fig. 1. Clinical and imaging data flow from the acquisition sites into separate clinical and imaging databases. Quality assessments and preprocessed images are generated by the imaging cores and returned to the central archive, where image analysts obtain, process, and return to the archive further derived image data and results.

deidentification, encrypted data transmission, database population, secure storage of the image files and metadata, and tracking of data accesses. The image archiving portion of the system is both robust and simple, with new users requiring little, if any, training. Key system components supporting the process of archiving raw data are:

1. The subject identifier is validated against a set of acceptable, site-specific identifiers.
2. Potentially patient-identifying information is removed or replaced. Raw image data are encoded in the digital imaging and communications in medicine (DICOM), emission computer-assisted tomography (ECAT), high resolution research tomograph (HRRT) file formats, from different scanner manufacturers and models (eg, Siemens Symphony [Siemens Corporation, Oxfordshire, Oxford, UK], GE Signa Excite [GE Healthcare, Waukesha, WI, USA], Philips Intera [Philips Healthcare, Latham, NY, USA]). The Java applet deidentification engine is customized for each of the image file formats deemed acceptable by the ADNI imaging cores, and any files not of an acceptable format are bypassed. Because the applet is sent to the upload site, all deidentification takes place at the acquisition site and no identifying information is transmitted.
3. Images are checked to see that they look appropriate for the type of upload. Phantom images uploaded under a patient identifier are flagged and removed from the upload set. This check is accomplished using a classifier that has been trained to identify human and phantom images.

4. Image files are transferred encrypted (HTTPS [Hypertext Transfer Protocol Secure]) to the repository in compliance with patient-privacy regulations.
5. Metadata elements are extracted from the image files and inserted into the database to support optimal storage and access. Customized database mappings were constructed for the various image file formats to provide consistency across scanners and image file formats.
6. Newly received images are placed into quarantine status, and the images are queued for those charged with performing MR and PET quality assessment.
7. Quality assessment results are imported from an external database and applied to the quarantined images. Images passing quality assessment are made available and images not passing quality control tagged as failing quality control.

Once raw data undergo quality assessment and are released from quarantine, they become immediately available to authorized users.

Processed image data
Preprocessed images are the recommended common set for analysis. The goals of preprocessing are to produce data standardized across site and scanner and with certain image artifacts corrected. Usability of processed data for further analysis requires an understanding of the data provenance, or information about the origin and subsequent processing applied to a set of data.

To provide almost immediate access to preprocessed data in a manner that preserved the relationship between the raw and preprocessed images and that captured processing provenance, we use an extended markup language (XML) schema that defines required metadata elements as well as standardized taxonomies. The system supports uploading large batches of preprocessed images in a single session with minimal interaction required by the person performing the upload. A key aspect of this process is agreement on the definitions of provenance metadata descriptors. Using standardized terms to describe processing minimizes variability and aids investigators in gaining an unambiguous interpretation of the data.

Preprocessed images are uploaded by the quality-control sites on a continuous basis. To minimize duplicate analyses, an automated data collection component was implemented whereby newly uploaded preprocessed scans are placed into predefined, shared data collections. These shared collections, organized by patient diagnostic group (normal control, mild cognitive impairment [MCI], AD) and visit (baseline, 6-month, and so forth), together with a redesigned user interface (Fig. 2) that clearly indicates which

images have not previously been downloaded, greatly reduce the time and effort needed to obtain new data. The same process may be used for postprocessed data, allowing analysts to share processing protocols via descriptive information contained in the XML metadata files.

DATA INTEGRATION

A subset of data from the clinical database is also integrated into the IDA to support richer multimodal queries across the combined set (Fig. 3). The selection of the initial set of clinical data elements was based on user surveys in which participants identified the elements they believed would be most useful in supporting their investigations. Because the clinical data originate in an external database, automated methods for obtaining and integrating the external data also validate and synchronize the data from the 2 sources and ensure that data from the same subject visit are combined.

INFRASTRUCTURE MECHANICS

A robust and reliable infrastructure is a necessity for supporting a resource intended to serve

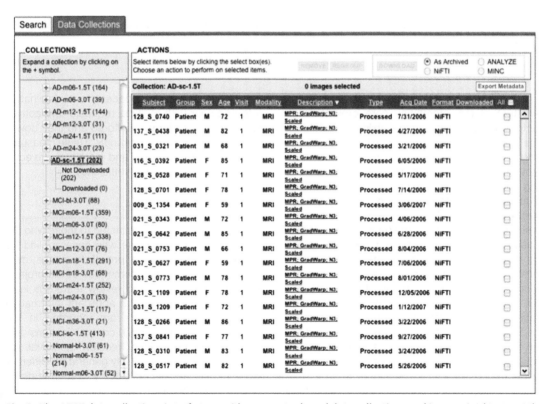

Fig. 2. The ADNI data collections interface provides access to shared data collections and is organized to meet the workflow needs of the analysts. The ability to easily select only images not previously downloaded by the user saves time and effort.

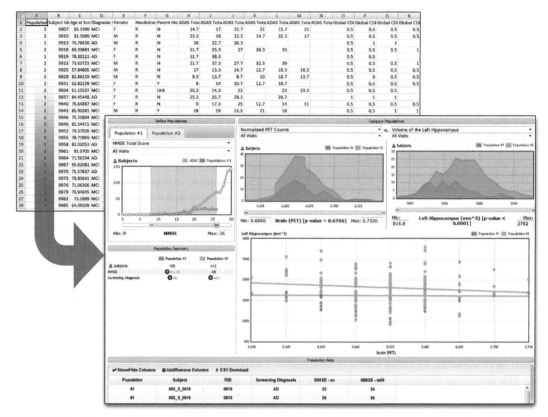

Fig. 3. This interface enables creation of groups from complex queries and comparison in a variety of graphical formats.

a global scientific community. The hardware infrastructure of the informatics core provides high performance, security, and reliability at each level. The fault-tolerant network infrastructure has no single points of failure. A firewall appliance protects and segments the network traffic, permitting only authorized ingress and egress. Multiple redundant database, application, and Web servers ensure service continuity in the event of a single system failure and also provide improved performance through load balancing of requests across the multiple machines. To augment the network-based security practices and to ensure compliance with privacy requirements, the servers use SSL (secure sockets layer) encryption for all data transfers. Posttransfer redundancy checking on the files is performed to guarantee the integrity of the data. Backup systems are designed to ensure data integrity and to protect data in the event of catastrophic failure.

ADNI policy requires participating sites to upload new data within 24 hours of acquisition. To prevent performance degradation, the application servers are divided by upload/download functionality. To prevent a single downloader from dominating a Web server with multiple requests, the activity of each downloader is monitored and their download rate is throttled accordingly. These measures help to ensure ADNI data and resources are equitably shared with maximal efficiency.

Data Access and Security

Access to ADNI data is restricted to those who are site participants and those who have applied for access and received approval from the data sharing and publication committee of the project. An online application and review feature is integrated into the IDA so that applicant information and committee decisions are recorded in the database and the e-mail communications acknowledging application receipt, approval, or disapproval are automatically generated. Different levels of user access control the system features available to an individual. All data uploads, changes, and deletions are logged.

More than 100,000 image data sets (more than 5 million files) and related clinical, imaging, biomarker, and genetic data sets are available to approved investigators. More than 1 million downloads of raw, preprocessed, and postprocessed scans have been provided. Clinical, biomarker, image analysis results, and genetic data have been downloaded more than 5000 times. Data download activity has increased annually since the data first became available in 2007. There are users from across the globe accessing the archive around the clock.

Data Management

There are data user management tools for reviewing data use applications, managing manuscript submissions, and sending notifications to investigators whose annual ADNI update is due. There is also a set of project summary tools that support interactive views of upload and download activities by site, user, and time period, and provide exports of these. Other information, documents, and resources geared toward apprising investigators about the status of the study and data available in the archive are provided through the ADNI Web site (http://adni.loni.ucla.edu/).

The informatics core provides a mechanism to distribute and share data, results, and information not only among the project participants but also the scientific community at large. This informatics model enables a more extensive array of analytical strategies and approaches to interpreting these data. These dissemination aspects of ADNI are among the most important to the success of the project. The databasing, querying, examination, and processing of data sets from multiple subjects necessitate efficient and intuitive interfaces, responsive answers to searches, coupled analyses workflows, and comprehensive provenance with a view toward promoting independent reanalysis and study replication. A new interface enabling interactive data mining and analyses has been developed (see **Fig. 3**).

Lessons Learned by the ADNI Informatics Core

Successful informatics solutions must build a trust with the communities they seek to serve and provide dependable services and open policies to researchers. Several factors contribute to database usefulness, including whether it contains viable data and these are accompanied by a detailed description of their acquisition (eg, metadata); whether the database is well organized and the user interface is easy to navigate; whether the data are derived versions of raw data or the raw data themselves; the manner in which the database addresses the sociologic and bureaucratic issues that can be associated with data

sharing; whether it has a policy in place to ensure that requesting investigators give proper attribution to the original collectors of the data; and the efficiency of secure data transactions. These systems must provide flexible methods for data description and relationships among various metadata characteristics. Moreover, those systems that have been specifically designed to serve a large and diverse audience with a variety of needs and that possess the qualities described earlier represent the types of databases that can have the greatest benefit to scientists looking to study a disease, assess new methods, examine previously published data, or explore novel ideas using the data.

Lessons learned to date by the informatics core include the following principles: (1) the data archive information must be open and unrestricted; (2) the database must be transparent in terms of activity and content; (3) the duties and responsibilities of stakeholder individuals and institutions must be clearly and precisely specified; (4) technical and semantic interoperability between the database and other online resources (data and analyses) is the optimal approach; (5) clear curation systems governing quality control, data validation, authentication, and authorization must be in place; (6) the systems must be operationally efficient and flexible; (7) clear policies of respect for intellectual property and other ethical and legal requirements must be in place before access is allowed; (8) management accountability and authority are obligatory; (9) a solid technological architecture and supporting expertise are essential; (10) systems for user support must be reliable; (11) Health Insurance Portability and Accountability Act compliance must be thorough and ever-adaptable to changes in regulatory and statutory fashion.

Scientific Advances and Future Vision of ADNI

With a current enrollment and ongoing longitudinal follow-up of more than 800 individuals with MCI and mild AD, as well as cognitively normal older individuals, across 57 project implementation sites in North America, the ADNI databases encompass a substantial convergence of data from medical evaluations; clinical, cognitive, functional, and behavioral assessments; biochemical analytics; structural and functional neuroimages; and genetic assessments. New and important insights into the neurobiology of the AD spectrum have emerged from the collective analytical effort,[27,31] particularly, as intended, in the realm of biomarkers as indirect measures or diagnostics of disease severity and as dynamic trackers of disease progression, with attendant implications for treatment trial design with respect to sample size and statistical powering as well as subject stratification.[28,32,33]

ADNI investigators have used multiple imaging biomarkers to quantify disease progression and measure various aspects of AD disease. These biomarkers include PET for amyloid, fluorodeoxyglucose (FDG) PET for metabolic decline, and MR imaging for brain atrophy, as well as risk factors that influence these measures (eg, apolipoprotein E [ApoE], cardiovascular risks).[2,34–38] Patients with MCI and AD experience progressive brain atrophy, and this has proved an especially fertile area for investigators to illuminate predictability in regional and temporal patterns of damage through neuroimaging because patients are followed longitudinally through disease progression and the trajectory of neurodegeneration is documented through imaging. In vivo measures and quantification of subregional atrophy, such as changes in cortical thickness or structure volume, hold great promise of improved diagnosis as well as assessment of the neuroprotective effects of newly developed therapies undergoing early-phase and late-phase trials.[39–41] Through 3D mapping of gray matter atrophy, ADNI researchers have found that cortical areas affected earlier in the disease process are more severely damaged than those that are affected late, suggesting that structural MR imaging is reliable not only as an in vivo disease-tracking technique but also may prove useful in evaluating disease-modifying therapies.[42,43] ADNI MR imaging metrics indicate that degree of neurodegeneration of medial temporal structures is a reliable antecedent imaging marker of imminent conversion from MCI to AD, with decreased hippocampal volume as the most robust marker. Validation of imaging biomarkers is thus critical because they can render clinical trials of disease-modifying agents more efficacious by identifying individuals who are at highest risk for progression to AD.[44]

ADNI data have been used in the elucidation of associations between various imaging, cerebrospinal fluid (CSF), genetic, and clinical measures in different cohorts. ADNI investigators have examined brain morphometric changes alone that occur during disease progression using cross-sectional and longitudinal MR imaging data.

Morphometry
Specific morphometric measures such as regional cortical thickness provide excellent sensitivity to group differences. In a cross-sectional study of normal controls and individuals with MCI or AD, differences were found mostly in the hippocampus

and entorhinal cortex, which had the largest effect sizes, along with other temporal regions, the temporal horn of the lateral ventricle, rostral posterior cingulated, and some parietal and frontal regions.[45] Additional atrophy was seen in patients with AD relative to controls in the inferior parietal, banks of the superior temporal sulcus, retrosplenial, and some frontal regions. Similar results were shown by Karow and colleagues.[46] However, the trajectories of change over the course of the disease vary.[45] Mesial and temporal regions showed a linear rate of atrophy through both MCI stages to AD, whereas the lateral temporal middle gyrus, retrosplenial, inferior parietal, and rostral midfrontal cortices showed accelerated atrophy later in the disease.

Leung and colleagues[47] also found higher rates of hippocampal atrophy in MCI converters to AD than nonconverters. McDonald and colleagues[48] examined regional rates of neocortical atrophy in 2 groups of patients with MCI with different degrees of impairment. As the disease progressed, atrophy migrated from the medial and inferior lateral temporal, inferior parietal, and posterior cingulate to the superior parietal, prefrontal, and lateral occipital cortex and then to the anterior cingulate cortex. The least-impaired patients with MCI showed the greatest rates of atrophy in the medial temporal cortex. Using a variety of approaches these findings are consistent. Hua and colleagues[49] and Leow and colleagues[20] all used tensor-based morphology (TBM), producing annualized 3D maps of structural changes. Schuff and colleagues[50] focused on changes in hippocampal volume, and McEvoy and colleagues[51] calculated an atrophy score based on regions of interest most associated with AD atrophy. Collectively, these studies showed atrophy spreading from the medial temporal lobe to the parietal, occipital, and frontal lobes over the course of the disease, with patients with MCI in general having a more anatomically restricted AD-like pattern of change. Individuals with MCI who converted to AD within the time frame of the study had a more AD-like pattern of atrophy.

Shape
Beyond simple volumetric analysis, is the assessment of changes in the shape of regions of interest. Qiu and colleagues[52] used diffeomorphic metric mapping to reveal that the anterior segment of the hippocampus and the basolateral complex of the amygdala had the most surface-inward deformation in patients with MCI or AD, coupled with a complementary outward deformation in the lateral ventricles. Similarly, Apostolova and colleagues[53] found enlargement of the lateral ventricles with disease progression.

Relation to cognition

It has been well established that structures within the temporal lobe decline in AD. Because of their critical role in the formation of memories, it is one of the first functions to be measurably affected in AD. Within the temporal lobe, hippocampal atrophy is a common structural biomarker because it is among the earliest to degenerate in AD. Leow and colleagues[20] found a strong association between several cognitive scores and temporal lobe atrophy in patients with MCI. Similarly, Morra and colleagues[54] found that bilateral hippocampal atrophy at baseline was strongly correlated with the Mini Mental State Examination (MMSE). Using TBM, Hua and colleagues[19] found that baseline temporal lobe atrophy was associated with both baseline and change in the Clinical Dementia Rating Scale-Sum of the Boxes score in patients with MCI or AD, but with change in the MMSE only in the AD group, providing further evidence for the acceleration of atrophic change with disease progression.

Genetics

Morra and colleagues,[55] Wolz and colleagues,[56] Hua and colleagues,[49] and Risacher and colleagues[57] all found that carriers of the APOE4 allele had higher rates of hippocampal atrophy than noncarriers. Vemuri and colleagues[58] also found that the APOE4 genotype contributed to MR imaging atrophy. Hua and colleagues[49] found that the APOE4 allele had a dose-dependent detrimental risk, with greater atrophy in the hippocampus and temporal lobe in homozygotes than heterozygotes in MCI and AD groups. The recently identified AD risk allele, GRIN2b, was associated with higher rates of temporal lobe atrophy in the pooled group, but more weakly than APOE4.[59] Other unidentified genetic risk factors likely contribute to AD, with epidemiologic studies suggesting that maternal history of the disease increases the risk of developing AD.

Other interesting associations

Using the related method of TBM, Ho and colleagues[60] created regional maps of changes in brain tissue and used the resulting Jacobian values to represent brain tissue excess or deficit relative to a template. These investigators found that lower brain volume in the frontal, parietal, occipital, and temporal lobes was associated with higher body mass index (BMI, calculated as weight in kilograms divided by the square of height in meters) in patients with MCI or AD and that ventricular expansion correlated with higher BMI in patients with AD but not MCI.

PET

FDG-PET has been used by several groups to investigate relationships between cerebral glucose hypometabolism and other factors, including cognitive measures and CSF biomarkers in cohorts with MCI or AD. Wu and colleagues[61] showed hypometabolic rates in posterior cingulate/precuneus and parietotemporal regions. Chen and colleagues[62] investigated declines in cerebral metabolic rate, glucose (CMRgl) in statistically predefined regions of interest associated with AD over 12 months in the ADNI cohort and found significant changes in MCI and AD groups compared with controls bilaterally in the posterior cingulate, medial and lateral parietal, medial and lateral temporal, frontal, and occipital cortex. These, and many other, studies support the use of glucose metabolism as a sensitive measure of cognition in AD.

SUMMARY

Given the vagaries of disease modification and of what will eventually prove a valid, reliable, and compelling empiric basis for distinguishing between true disease modification and symptomatic treatment effects, ADNI investigators are bringing multimodal neuroimaging techniques to the cutting edge of usefulness as dynamic biomarkers, sensitive to disease state and progression across different stages.[18,33,63] From here, the next step is neuroimages as reliable treatment trial end points and clinical intervention outcomes with respect to longitudinal changes in brain volume, enhancing both the feasibility and the cost efficiencies of trials through improved signal detection of novel treatments.[64] Inasmuch as AD is a devastating neurodegenerative disease against which no effective treatment is known, ADNI and similar discovery initiatives worldwide give solid hope for the future in patient care.

ACKNOWLEDGMENTS

The original work was primarily funded by the ADNI (Principal Investigator: Michael Weiner; National Institutes of Health (NIH) grant number U01 AG024904). ADNI is funded by the National Institute of Aging, the National Institute of Biomedical Imaging and Bioengineering, and the Foundation for the National Institutes of Health, through generous contributions from the following companies and organizations: Pfizer Inc, Wyeth Research, Bristol-Myers Squibb, Eli Lilly and Company, GlaxoSmithKline, Merck & Co Inc, AstraZeneca AB, Novartis Pharmaceuticals Corporation, the Alzheimer's Association, Eisai Global Clinical Development, Elan Corporation plc, Forest Laboratories, and the Institute for the Study of

Aging, with participation from the US Food and Drug Administration. The grantee organization is the Northern California Institute for Research and Education, and the study is coordinated by the Alzheimer's Disease Cooperative Study at the University of California, San Diego. This study was also supported by grant P41 RR013642 from the National Center for Research Resources, NIH. The author would also like to acknowledge a deep appreciation to Franci Duitch for her editorial contributions.

REFERENCES

1. Evans AC. Large-scale morphometric analysis of neuroanatomy and neuropathology. Anat Embryol 2005;210(5–6):439–46.
2. Frisoni GB, Redolfi A, Manset D, et al. Virtual imaging laboratories for marker discovery in neurodegenerative diseases. Nat Rev Neurol 2011;7(8):429–38.
3. Toga AW. Guest editorial: a vision of computational anatomy. Biomed Comput Rev 2009;5(3):1.
4. Joshi SH, Horn JD, Toga AW. Interactive exploration of neuroanatomical meta-spaces. Front Neuroinform 2009;3:38.
5. Dinov I, Lozev K, Petrosyan P, et al. Neuroimaging study designs, computational analyses and data provenance using the LONI pipeline. PloS One 2010;5(9):pii:e13070.
6. Dinov ID, Van Horn JD, Lozev KM, et al . Efficient, distributed and interactive neuroimaging data analysis using the LONI Pipeline. Front Neuroinform 2009;3:22.
7. Shattuck DW, Prasad G, Mirza M, et al. Online resource for validation of brain segmentation methods. Neuroimage 2009;45(2):431–9.
8. Shi Y, Lai R, Morra JH, et al. Robust surface reconstruction via Laplace-Beltrami eigen-projection and boundary deformation. IEEE Trans Med Imaging 2010;29(12):2009–22.
9. Cohen JR, Asarnow RF, Sabb FW, et al. Decoding continuous variables from neuroimaging data: basic and clinical applications. Front Neurosci 2011;5:75.
10. Pievani M, de Haan W, Wu T, et al. Functional network disruption in the degenerative dementias. Lancet Neurol 2011;10(9):829–43.
11. Toga AW, Thompson PM, Mori S, et al. Towards multimodal atlases of the human brain. Nat Rev Neurol 2006;7(12):952–66.
12. Van Horn JD, Toga AW. Multisite neuroimaging trials. Curr Opin Neurol 2009;22(4):370–8.
13. Sporns O. The human connectome: a complex network. Ann N Y Acad Sci 2011;1224(1):109–25.
14. Biswal BB, Mennes M, Zuo XN, et al. Toward discovery science of human brain function. Proc Natl Acad Sci U S A 2010;107(10):4734–9.
15. Mackenzie-Graham AJ, Van Horn JD, Woods RP, et al. Provenance in neuroimaging. Neuroimage 2008;42(1):178–95.
16. Toga AW, Thompson PM. What is where and why it is important. Neuroimage 2007;37(4):1045–9 [discussion: 1066–8].
17. Zhang D, Wang Y, Zhou L, et al. Multimodal classification of Alzheimer's disease and mild cognitive impairment. Neuroimage 2011;55(3):856–67.
18. Ewers M, Frisoni GB, Teipel SJ, et al. Staging Alzheimer's disease progression with multimodality neuroimaging. Prog Neurobiol 2011;95(4):535–46.
19. Hua X, Leow AD, Lee S, et al. 3D characterization of brain atrophy in Alzheimer's disease and mild cognitive impairment using tensor-based morphometry. Neuroimage 2008;41(1):19–34.
20. Leow AD, Yanovsky I, Parikshak N, et al. Alzheimer's disease neuroimaging initiative: a one-year follow up study using tensor-based morphometry correlating degenerative rates, biomarkers and cognition. Neuroimage 2009;45(3):645–55.
21. Madsen SK, Ho AJ, Hua X, et al. 3D maps localize caudate nucleus atrophy in 400 Alzheimer's disease, mild cognitive impairment, and healthy elderly subjects. Neurobiol Aging 2010;31(8):1312–25.
22. Thompson PM, Hayashi KM, Dutton RA, et al. Tracking Alzheimer's disease. Ann N Y Acad Sci 2007;1097:183–214.
23. Morra JH, Tu Z, Apostolova LG, et al. Automated 3D mapping of hippocampal atrophy and its clinical correlates in 400 subjects with Alzheimer's disease, mild cognitive impairment, and elderly controls. Hum Brain Mapp 2009;30(9):2766–88.
24. Westman E, Simmons A, Muehlboeck JS, et al. AddNeuroMed and ADNI: similar patterns of Alzheimer's atrophy and automated MRI classification accuracy in Europe and North America. Neuroimage 2011;58(3):818–28.
25. Sakoglu Ü, Upadhyay J, Chin CL, et al. Paradigm shift in translational neuroimaging of CNS disorders. Biochem Pharmacol 2011;81(12):1374–87.
26. Schumann G, Loth E, Banaschewski T, et al. The IMAGEN study: reinforcement-related behaviour in normal brain function and psychopathology. Mol Psychiatry 2010;15(12):1128–39.
27. Aisen PS, Petersen RC, Donohue MC, et al. Clinical core of the Alzheimer's disease neuroimaging initiative: progress and plans. Alzheimers Dement 2010;6(3):239–46.
28. Beckett LA, Harvey DJ, Gamst A, et al. The Alzheimer's disease neuroimaging initiative: annual change in biomarkers and clinical outcomes. Alzheimers Dement 2010;6(3):257–64.
29. Petersen RC, Aisen PS, Beckett LA, et al. Alzheimer's disease neuroimaging initiative (ADNI): clinical characterization. Neurology 2010;74(3):201–9.

30. Toga AW, Crawford KL. The informatics core of the Alzheimer's Disease Neuroimaging Initiative. Alzheimers Dement 2010;6(3):247–56.

31. Weiner MW, Aisen PS, Jack CR Jr, et al. The Alzheimer's disease neuroimaging initiative: progress report and future plans. Alzheimers Dement 2010; 6(3):202–11.

32. Thal LJ, Kantarci K, Reiman EM, et al. The role of biomarkers in clinical trials for Alzheimer disease. Alzheimer Dis Assoc Disord 2006;20(1):6–15.

33. Cavedo E, Frisoni GB. The dynamic marker hypothesis of Alzheimer's disease and its implications for clinical imaging. Q J Nucl Med Mol Imaging 2011; 55(3):237–49.

34. Jagust WJ, Bandy D, Chen K, et al. The Alzheimer's disease neuroimaging initiative positron emission tomography core. Alzheimers Dement 2010;6(3): 221–9.

35. Kohannim O, Hua X, Hibar DP, et al. Boosting power for clinical trials using classifiers based on multiple biomarkers. Neurobiol Aging 2010;31(8): 1429–42.

36. Petersen RC. Alzheimer's disease: progress in prediction. Lancet Neurol 2010;9(1):4–5.

37. Jack CR Jr, Knopman DS, Jagust WJ, et al. Hypothetical model of dynamic biomarkers of the Alzheimer's pathological cascade. Lancet Neurol 2010;9(1):119–28.

38. Jack CR Jr, Wiste HJ, Vemuri P, et al. Brain beta-amyloid measures and magnetic resonance imaging atrophy both predict time-to-progression from mild cognitive impairment to Alzheimer's disease. Brain 2010;133(11):3336–48.

39. Hampel H, Shen Y, Walsh DM, et al. Biological markers of amyloid beta-related mechanisms in Alzheimer's disease. Exp Neurol 2010;223(2):334–46.

40. Hampel H, Wilcock G, Andrieu S, et al. Biomarkers for Alzheimer's disease therapeutic trials. Prog Neurobiol 2010;95(4):579–93.

41. Holland D, Brewer JB, Hagler DJ, et al. Subregional neuroanatomical change as a biomarker for Alzheimer's disease. Proc Natl Acad Sci U S A 2009; 106(49):20954–9.

42. Apostolova LG, Steiner CA, Akopyan GG, et al. Three-dimensional gray matter atrophy mapping in mild cognitive impairment and mild Alzheimer disease. Arch Neurol 2007;64(10):1489–95.

43. Apostolova LG, Thompson PM, Green AE, et al. 3D comparison of low, intermediate, and advanced hippocampal atrophy in MCI. Hum Brain Mapp 2010;31(5):786–97.

44. Risacher SL, Saykin AJ, West JD, et al. Baseline MRI predictors of conversion from MCI to probable AD in the ADNI cohort. Curr Alzheimer Res 2009;6(4): 347–61.

45. Fennema-Notestine C, Hagler DJ Jr, McEvoy LK, et al. Structural MRI biomarkers for preclinical and mild Alzheimer's disease. Hum Brain Mapp 2009; 30(10):3238–53.

46. Karow DS, McEvoy LK, Fennema-Notestine C, et al. Relative capability of MR imaging and FDG PET to depict changes associated with prodromal and early Alzheimer disease. Radiology 2010;256(3): 932–42.

47. Leung KK, Barnes J, Ridgway GR, et al. Automated cross-sectional and longitudinal hippocampal volume measurement in mild cognitive impairment and Alzheimer's disease. Neuroimage 2010;51(4): 1345–59.

48. McDonald CR, McEvoy LK, Gharapetian L, et al. Regional rates of neocortical atrophy from normal aging to early Alzheimer disease. Neurology 2009; 73(6):457–65.

49. Hua X, Leow AD, Parikshak N, et al. Tensor-based morphometry as a neuroimaging biomarker for Alzheimer's disease: an MRI study of 676 AD, MCI, and normal subjects. Neuroimage 2008;43(3): 458–69.

50. Schuff N, Tosun D, Insel PS, et al. Nonlinear time course of brain volume loss in cognitively normal and impaired elders. Neurobiol Aging 2010. [Epub ahead of print].

51. McEvoy LK, Fennema-Notestine C, Roddey JC, et al. Alzheimer disease: quantitative structural neuroimaging for detection and prediction of clinical and structural changes in mild cognitive impairment. Radiology 2009;251(1):195–205.

52. Qiu A, Fennema-Notestine C, Dale AM, et al. Regional shape abnormalities in mild cognitive impairment and Alzheimer's disease. Neuroimage 2009;45(3):656–61.

53. Apostolova LG, Morra JH, Green AE, et al. Automated 3D mapping of baseline and 12-month associations between three verbal memory measures and hippocampal atrophy in 490 ADNI subjects. Neuroimage 2010;51(1):488–99.

54. Morra JH, Tu Z, Apostolova LG, et al. Validation of a fully automated 3D hippocampal segmentation method using subjects with Alzheimer's disease mild cognitive impairment, and elderly controls. Neuroimage 2008;43(1):59–68.

55. Morra JH, Tu Z, Apostolova LG, et al. Automated mapping of hippocampal atrophy in 1-year repeat MRI data from 490 subjects with Alzheimer's disease, mild cognitive impairment, and elderly controls. Neuroimage 2009;45(Suppl 1):S3–15.

56. Wolz R, Heckemann RA, Aljabar P, et al. Measurement of hippocampal atrophy using 4D graph-cut segmentation: application to ADNI. Neuroimage 2010;52(1):109–18.

57. Risacher SL, Shen L, West JD, et al. Longitudinal MRI atrophy biomarkers: relationship to conversion in the ADNI cohort. Neurobiol Aging 2010;31(8): 1401–18.

58. Vemuri P, Wiste HJ, Weigand SD, et al. Effect of apoli-poprotein E on biomarkers of amyloid load and neuronal pathology in Alzheimer disease. Ann Neurol 2010;67(3):308–16.

59. Hua X, Hibar DP, Lee S, et al. Sex and age differences in atrophic rates: an ADNI study with n=1368 MRI scans. Neurobiol Aging 2010;31(8):1463–80.

60. Ho AJ, Raji CA, Becker JT, et al. Obesity is linked with lower brain volume in 700 AD and MCI patients. Neurobiol Aging 2010;31(8):1326–39.

61. Wu X, Chen K, Yao L, et al. Assessing the reliability to detect cerebral hypometabolism in probable Alzheimer's disease and amnestic mild cognitive impairment. J Neurosci Methods 2010;192(2):277–85.

62. Chen K, Langbaum JB, Fleisher AS, et al. Twelve-month metabolic declines in probable Alzheimer's disease and amnestic mild cognitive impairment assessed using an empirically pre-defined statistical region-of-interest: findings from the Alzheimer's Disease Neuroimaging Initiative. Neuroimage 2010;51(2):654–64.

63. Ewers M, Sperling RA, Klunk WE, et al. Neuroimaging markers for the prediction and early diagnosis of Alzheimer's disease dementia. Trends Neurosci 2011;34(8):430–42.

64. Valenzuela M, Bartrés-Faz D, Beg F, et al. Neuro-imaging as endpoints in clinical trials: are we there yet? Perspective from the first Provence workshop. Mol Psychiatry 2011;16(11):1064–6.

Index

Note: Page numbers of article titles are in **boldface** type.

neuroimaging.theclinics.com

Index

Printed and bound by CPI Group (UK) Ltd, Croydon, CR0 4YY

03/10/2024

01040350-0006